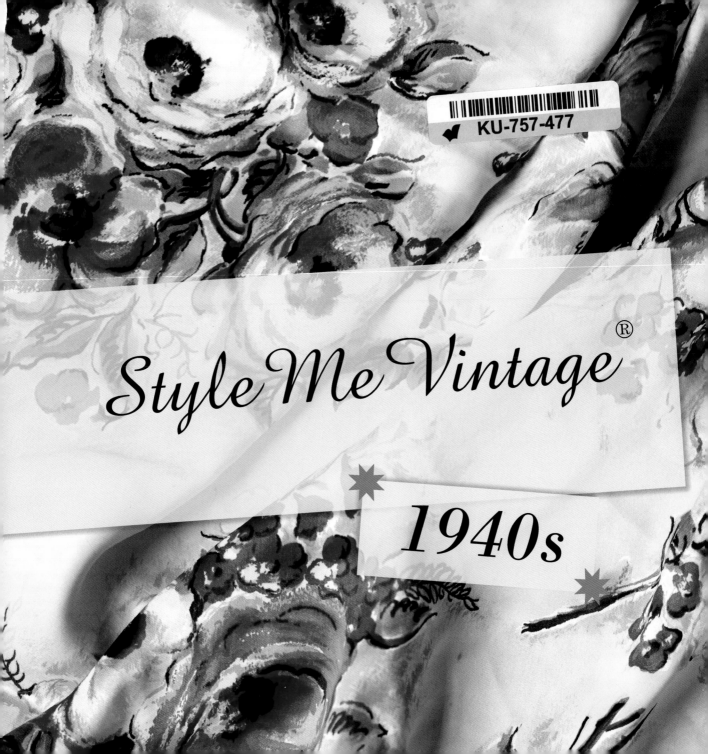

Style Me Vintage

1940s

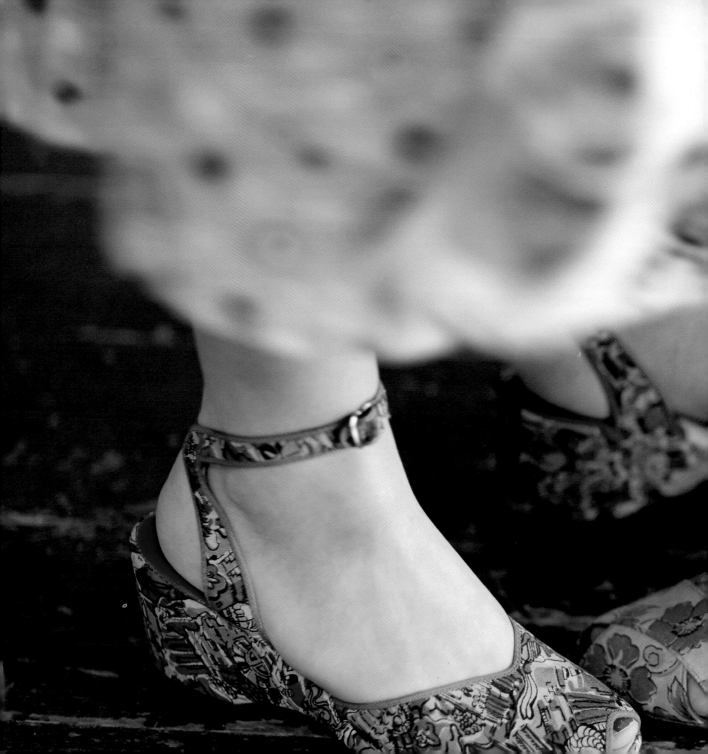

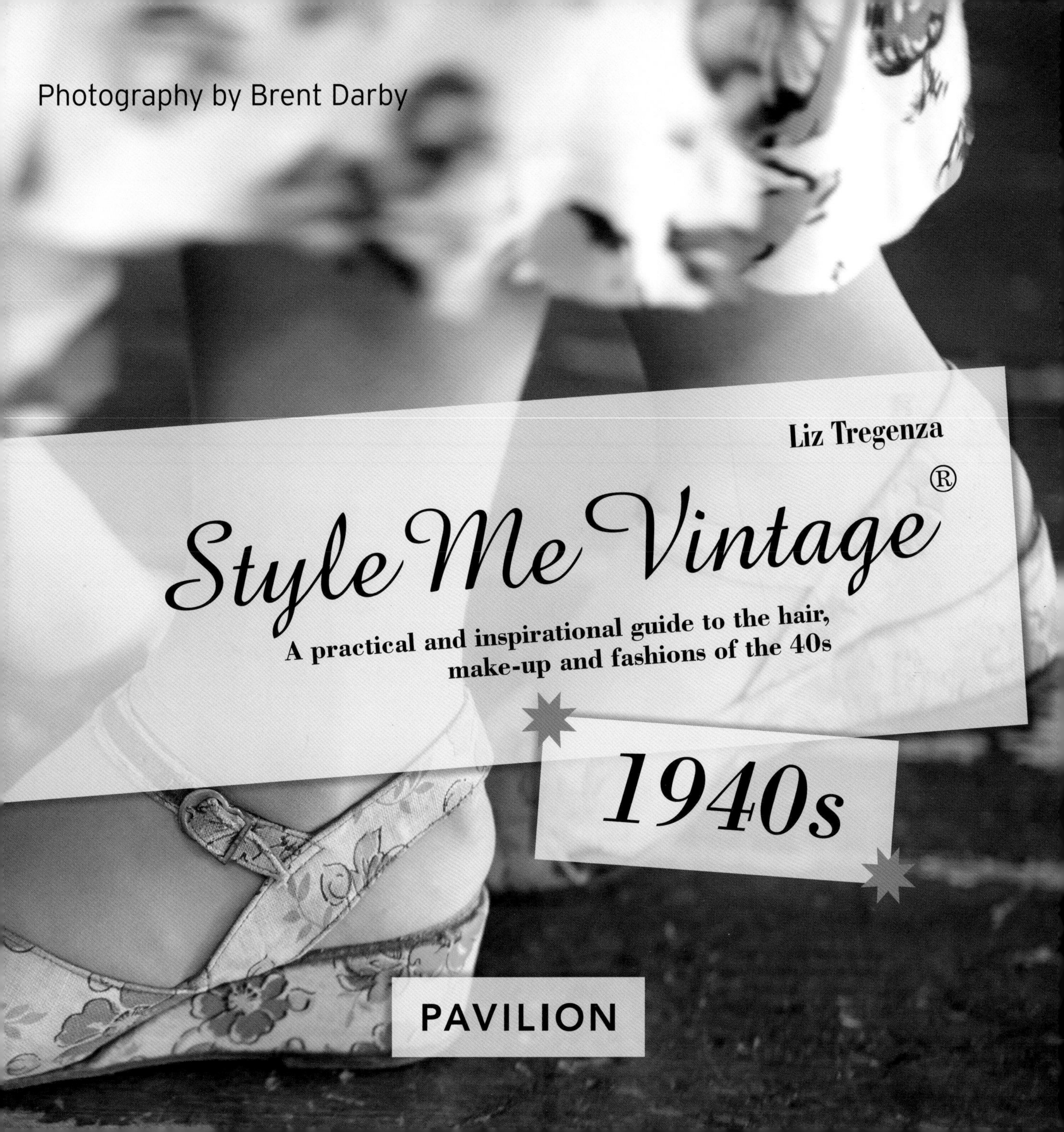

Photography by Brent Darby

Liz Tregenza

Style Me Vintage

A practical and inspirational guide to the hair,
make-up and fashions of the 40s

1940s

PAVILION

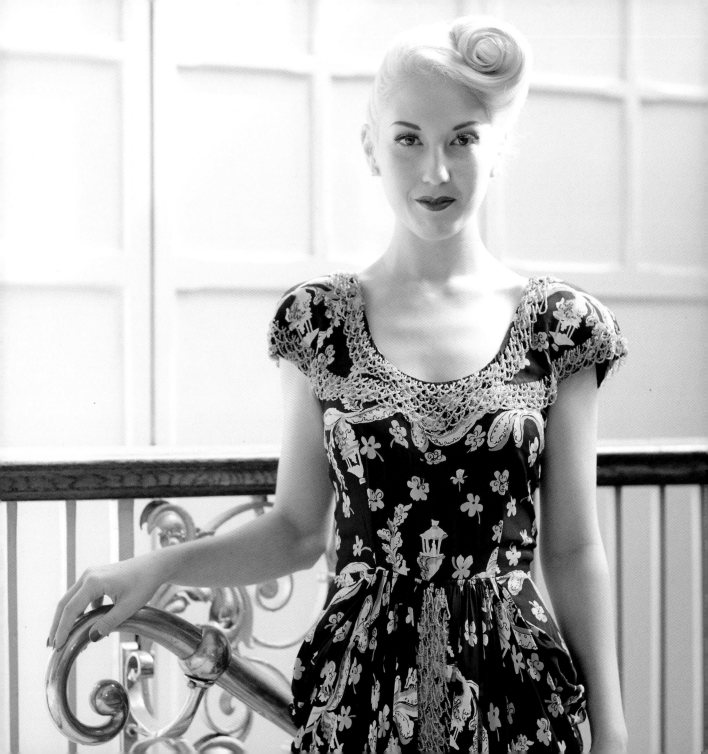

Contents

INTRODUCTION

Have you ever wanted to dress like a 40s Hollywood starlet? Or wondered how to execute the perfect Victory roll? Have you ever marvelled at how women kept themselves looking beautiful during wartime?

Whether you want to dress for a 40s evening soirée, the beach, or even for your wedding, from underwear to outerwear, from cosmetics to accessories, the tips are all here.

This book is a useful guide for vintage wearers and collectors alike. It doesn't matter if you are a vintage novice or a seasoned aficionado, there's something here for you. Interesting historical snippets are mixed in with useful and easy-to-master styling tips. I'll show you how to dress in original 40s garments, try out the style with later reproductions or just add a touch of authentic 40s to your outfit. I strongly believe that vintage looks should be simple to recreate – all the hair and make-up tips shown here are tried-and-tested favourites of mine.

At the back of the book I've also included a handy list of stockists of the best vintage and repro brands to help you source your own gems.

Right: One of my favourite family photos, my Nanna (right) stands with her friends Joyce and Tiny on the roof of the GEC building, May 1946.

Why a whole book about recreating the styles of the 1940s?

I have a personal fascination with the 1940s. My Nanna looked after me throughout my childhood and I was always riveted by her tales of yesteryear – whether it was stories of working during the Blitz in central London aged just fourteen, or her wonderful memories of beachtime frolics with her friends. Many of the original photographs you will see here are courtesy of my Nanna and give a real impression of the life of a young Londoner during the 40s.

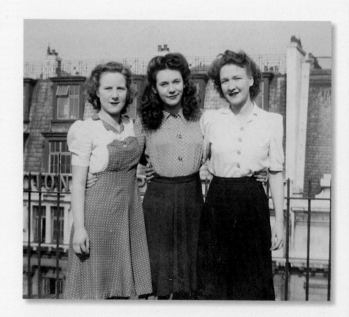

In my opinion the 1940s form an extraordinary decade in the history of women's clothing and style. This was a period of huge social and cultural change that affected every aspect of people's lives. The perceived role of women changed drastically during the decade and it was realised that they could perform jobs just as well as men could.

The way women dressed, styled their hair and wore their make-up altered because of the war. Female appearance was no longer simply about looking beautiful, it was also a matter of practicality and versatility. Clothes were made to last and hairstyles had to enable war work. Fashion and cosmetics did their bit for the war effort - they acted as a morale booster.

Sometimes the myth is propagated that fashion stopped during World War II. In Britain and the United States shortages, government regulations and wartime priorities brought slower changes in fashionable styles, yet fashion did not stop. Fashion changes between 1942 and 1946 occurred

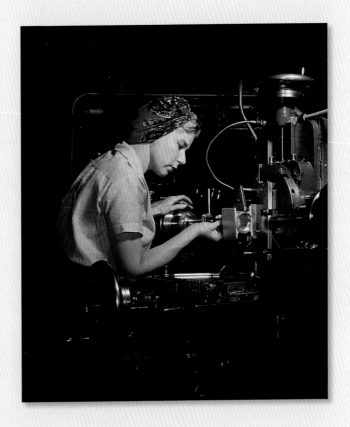

'You'll have fewer clothes because you have not the time, money or coupons to clutter your life with non-essentials [...] you'll have simpler clothes because in these days anything elaborate looks silly [...] you'll have better clothes because anything you buy will be chosen after long thought to last the duration – and beyond.' Vogue, November 1939

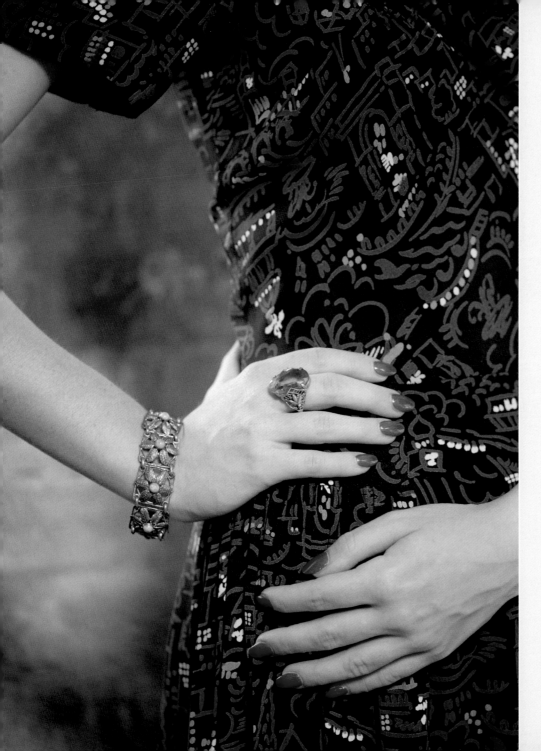

Left: I love a good novelty print. This rayon crêpe mid-1940s dress by Gracette is covered in a print of Parisian landmarks.

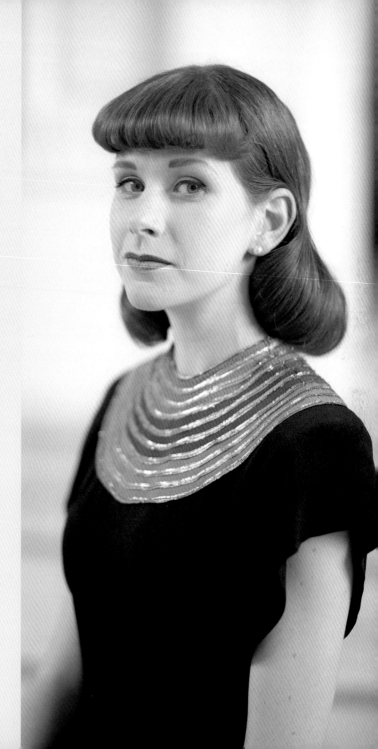

far more slowly than they had before the war, but decorative qualities still existed and women continued to update their wardrobes when coupons and funds allowed.

I wanted to dispel some misconceptions with this book. 1940s style isn't all victory rolls and drab, masculine suits brightened up with flashes of red lipstick. The 1940s was a hugely diverse decade in terms of style and, whatever your personal predilection – whether you like to dress in a feminine or masculine manner, wear your hair up or down, there is a facet of 1940s style to suit you.

The most important thing to remember though is to have fun – dressing in vintage should never be a chore, it should always be a pleasure. Use this book as a guide to help you hunt out those forgotten 40s treasures, make yourself feel like a 40s film star, or accurately recreate the swish of Dior's New Look.

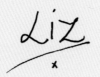

Make-up

'Cosmetics are as essential to a woman as a reasonable supply of tobacco is to a man.'

Mr. Henderson, Ministry of Supply, *Vogue*, August 1942

When most people think of 1940s make-up, it is the bold red lips of the decade that spring to mind. This, more than any other aspect of 1940s make-up, defines the era and was worn by women of all classes around the world. But there's more to 1940s make-up than just red lipstick.

The predominant make-up look of the 1940s was a natural, healthy one – pale to slightly tanned skin tones, gently pencilled brows, a thin coating of mascara, a dusting of pink to the cheeks, and all of this was topped off with a splash of that red lipstick.

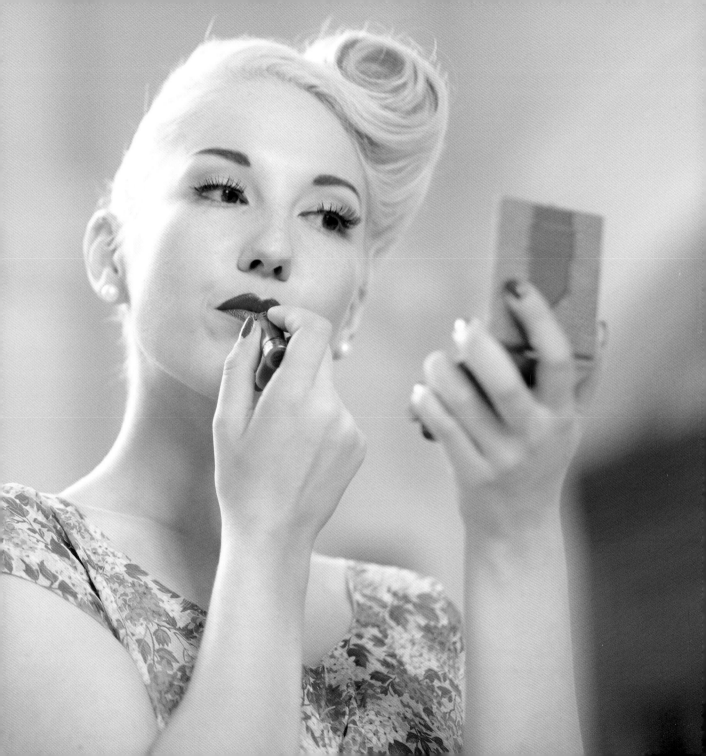

HISTORY

During the 1940s, as numerous cosmetics advertisements suggested, beauty was a woman's 'duty'. Make-up had a powerful effect on women and men alike during the war and women were actively encouraged to wear it. Wartime cosmetics advertisements presented powerful, strong women doing their bit for the war effort. A series of Yardley advertisements advocated that women should 'put your best face forward'. Make-up was seen as a morale booster, not only for the women who wore it, but also for the men who saw these glamorous women. Good looks and good morale were considered allies.

Wartime austerity however, particularly in Britain, limited women's cosmetics choices. In 1940 cosmetic production was cut to just 25% of pre-war levels. The metal used for casing cosmetics was needed for armaments. Petroleum and alcohol – essential ingredients for beauty products – were needed for the war effort too. Even soap was rationed, as glycerine was required for making munitions. It was far easier to purchase cosmetics in the United States than it was in Europe because the chemicals needed to produce them were not in such short supply.

Opposite: An advertisement for Yardley cosmetics, 1944.

Right: One of the most fashionable lip shapes of the 1940s was the Hunter's Bow (created by Max Factor for Joan Crawford in the 30s). This was a deep, rounded and full lip shape.

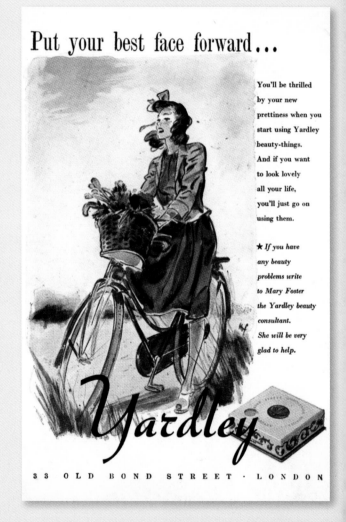

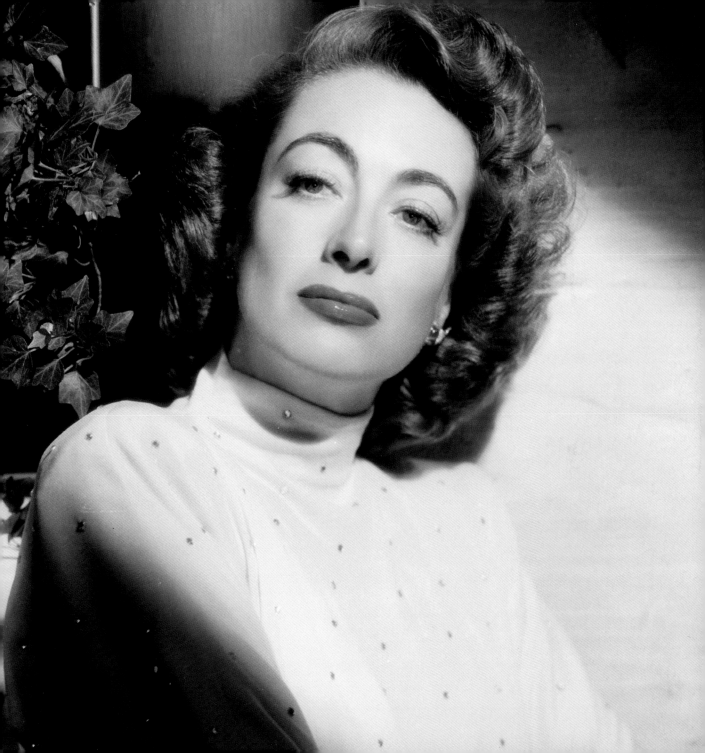

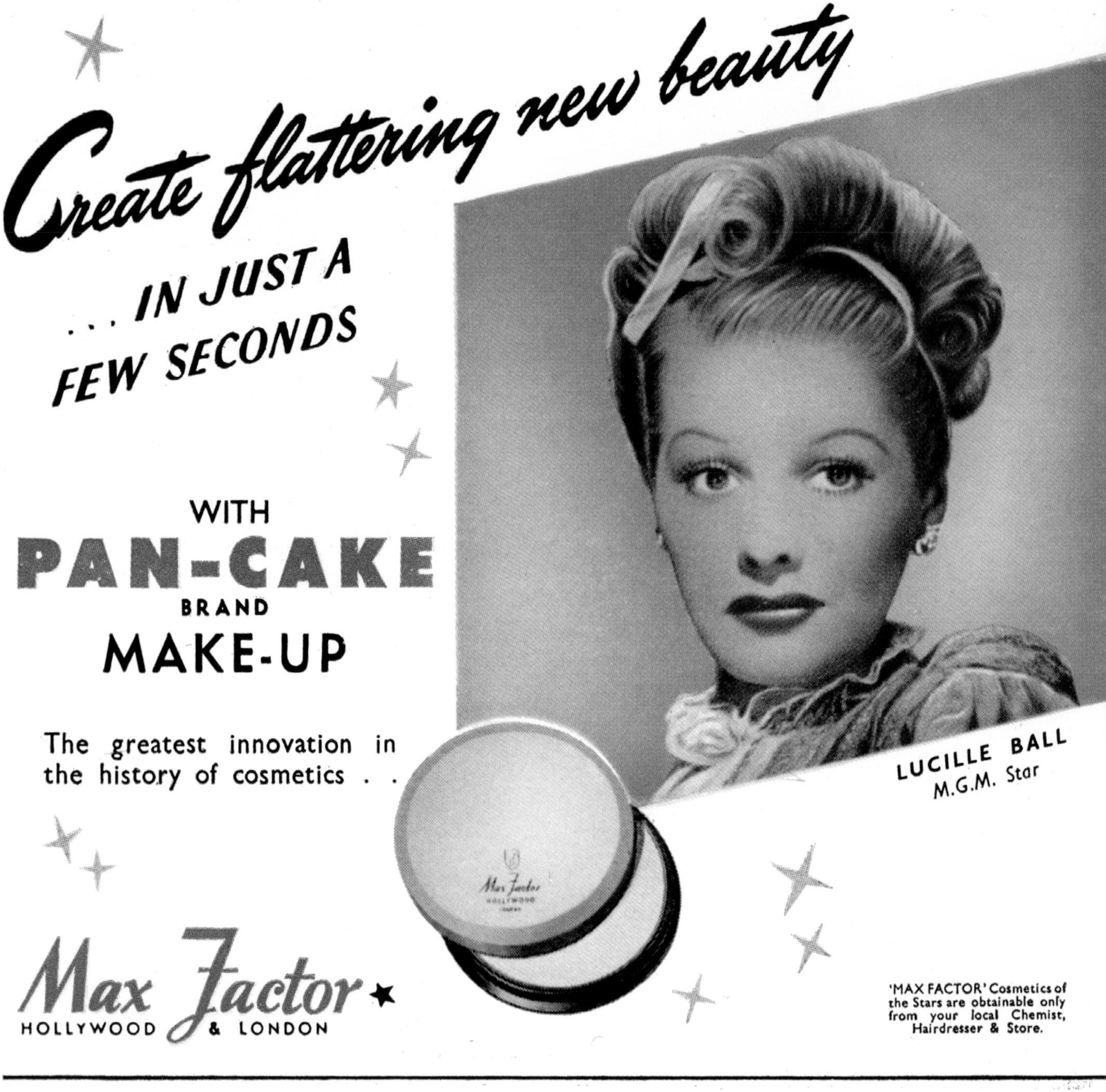

Create flattering new beauty
. . . IN JUST A
FEW SECONDS
WITH
PAN-CAKE
BRAND
MAKE-UP
The greatest innovation in the history of cosmetics . .
LUCILLE BALL
M.G.M. Star
Max Factor
HOLLYWOOD
Max Factor ★
HOLLYWOOD & LONDON
'MAX FACTOR' Cosmetics of the Stars are obtainable only from your local Chemist, Hairdresser & Store.

While cosmetics were harder to come by they were certainly still available. If you had the will, there was a way of procuring them. When cosmetic supplies reached the shops, word soon got out and women would queue for hours. Similarly, if you saw a lipstick – whether or not it was your colour – you bought it.

Cosmetics were often sold 'under the counter' or via the black market. Even old theatrical make-up was used when women became desperate – it was better than nothing.

Cosmetics firms got into the patriotic spirit. Cyclax introduced Auxiliary Red, while Elizabeth Arden produced lipstick and nail polish in Montezuma Red, said to be a perfect match to the scarf, arm insignia and hat cords on the American Marine Corps Women's Reserve uniforms. Post-war a number of companies produced celebratory cosmetics. Gala for example launched Red Bunting in 1946 'a rich red and blue toned lipstick'.

Left: Max Factor Pan-Cake advert from 1946.

Max Factor

Max Factor's Pan-Cake was for many a beauty staple. Max Factor had been one of the leading lights of Hollywood make-up design since 1914. His Pan-Cake make-up was initially developed for the silver screen (after the introduction of Technicolor). Once actresses saw the results of the foundation on screen they wanted to use it off screen too. Seeing an opportunity, Max Factor launched Pan-Cake to the public in the late 30s and it was a huge success. In 1948 the brand introduced Pan-Stik, a cream foundation in stick form housed in a twist up lipstick type container that women could pop in their handbags.

Make-up brands join the war effort

- Revlon made first-aid kits and dye markers for the US Navy.
- Cyclax , Elizabeth Arden, Helena Rubenstein and Max Factor all produced sun lotion and camouflage make-up to be used on the front line.
- Elizabeth Arden created scar creams for wounded soldiers.
- Stratton converted their lipstick machines to produce shell cases.

CREATING THE 1940S LOOK

Here I'll show you how to create a 1940s wartime face with some interesting historical facts along the way.

1.

2.

FOUNDATION

Foundation colours were geared towards creating a healthy glow. Often women used a warm foundation with a light pressed powder on top (fig. 1).

BLUSHER

In the 1940s what today we often call blusher was referred to as rouge. Rouge was sold in little pots of compressed powder - popular shades were peach, coral and bold pink. If women could not get hold of rouge many added a hint of colour to their cheeks with lipstick instead. Rouge in the 1940s was bright, creating a rosy glow. It was applied high on the cheekbone and then blended towards the temple (fig. 2).

EYES

During the war eyeshadow tended to be quite subtle, if women wore it at all. If you can't bear to be without eyeshadow it is best to wear one that creates a subtle and clean look - apply a nude shade to the lid, with a deep shade in the crease to accentuate the natural hollow.

To create a genuine wartime look use a thin coating of mascara. If you want more of a 'Hollywood glamour' look, a thick coating is appropriate. Mascara was quite different to the wand in a bottle we are used to today. It came in three formats; liquid, paste and solid cake, although the solid cake was the most often used and seemingly the most readily available. Women would spit onto the cake, work up the colour with a brush and apply the resulting mix to their eyelashes.

BROWS

The eyebrow of the 1940s was groomed, neat and carefully arched. It was far bigger and more defined than that of the 1920s and 1930s, but it was still not left to overgrow. Many women simply tamed their eyebrows with flour and water paste, but if you could get hold of an eyebrow pencil, eyebrows were arched or rounded.

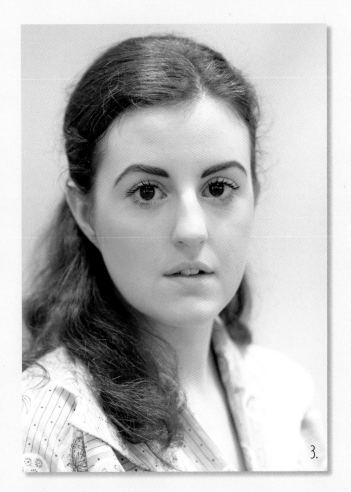
3.

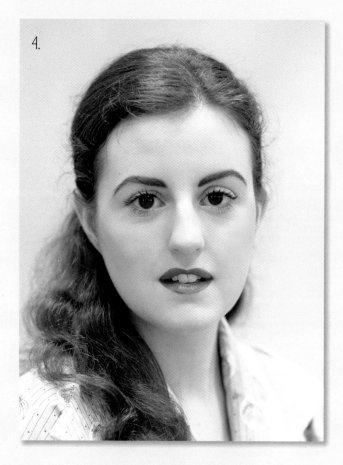

4.

LIPS

Red was the lipstick colour of the decade. There were a variety of reds available, but most women stuck to a strong pillarbox red. Lipsticks were matte, so if shine was required a dab of petroleum jelly was added.

Women tended to overdraw their lip line slightly in order to accentuate the full shape as much as possible. If you'd like to experiment with overdrawing your lip line, apply a light layer of foundation to your lips to blend over the natural lip before you start applying lip liner.

Lip pencils started to make their mark in the late 40s, but I would advocate using one when recreating any 40s look. This will help to define your mouth and prevent lipstick from straying too far. As a general rule it's best to line the mouth and also 'fill in' the lip with a liner in order to give the lipstick something to cling to.

Apply your lipstick with a lip brush - this will give you a smooth, even layer of lipstick. Make sure you blot the colour after the first application and apply a sprinkling of loose powder. Follow this up with a second application of colour, and then blot once more. The two layers of lipstick and subsequent blotting will improve the staying power of your lipstick.

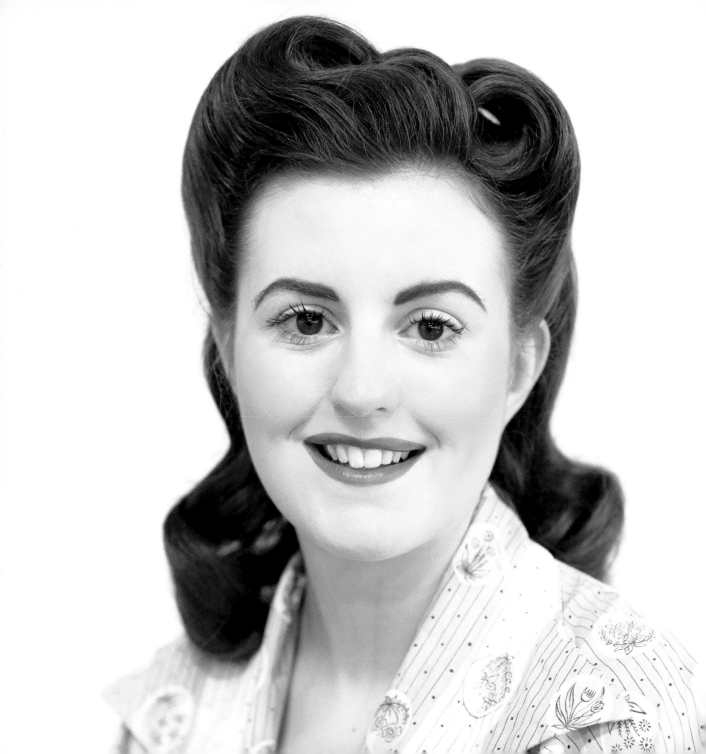

COMPACTS

At the outbreak of war, powder compacts with British armed forces insignia were produced for servicemen who wanted a gift for their sweethearts. Designs were often simple – a plain enamelled compact with a metal badge or regimental transfer applied to the centre. Yet metal was soon in short supply and the manufacture of metal compacts in Britain pretty much stopped during the war. British compacts during the war were therefore more often made in plastic.

America on the other hand continued to manufacture metal compacts throughout the war. Numerous brands produced inventive and ingenious novelty pieces during this period. For example Volupté produced compacts in the shape of hands, apples and even dressing tables!

Popular compact brands of the 40s
- Dorothy Gray
- Elgin
- Kigu
- Pygmalion
- Stratton
- Volupté
- Wadsworth

N.B. Most of these companies were still producing compacts after the 1940s.

TOP TIP
Vintage vanity items (especially compacts, perfume bottles and vanity cases) can add instant old-school glamour to any dressing table.

Right: A pot of bright pink Heather rogue and a triple vanity compact. The compact, a 'Swashbuckle' design, was produced by American brand Dorothy Gray between 1942 and 1948.

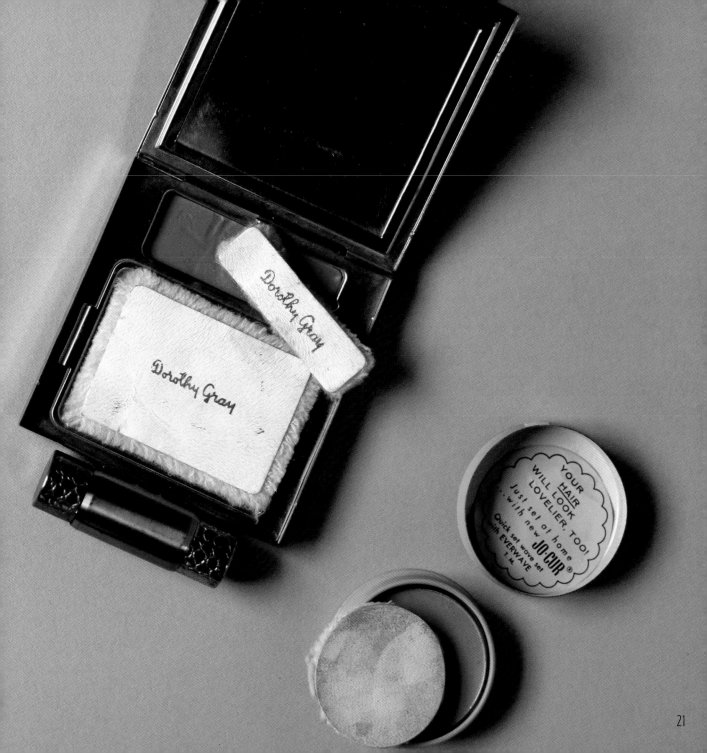

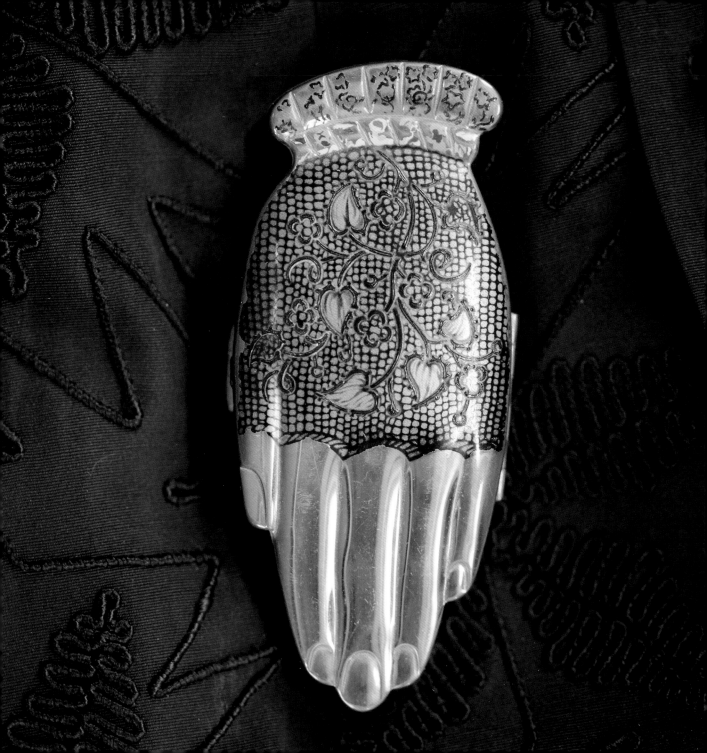

SHORTAGES AND ALTERNATIVES

With cosmetics in short supply during the war, women went to great lengths to ensure they could still look beautiful. Here are some of my favourite (if somewhat odd) alternatives:

- Burnt cork or boot polish – mascara
- Cochineal or beetroot – lipstick
- Bicarbonate of soda – deodorant
- Table salt – toothpaste
- Lead pencil – eyebrow pencil
- Pumice stone – razor
- Sooty residue mixed with petroleum jelly – eyeshadow
- Rose petals steeped in water – rouge
- Tiny amounts of lard and water – make-up remover

Owing to shortages lipsticks had to be eked out to their last vestige. Magazines advised women to scrape out the last of their old lipsticks, melt together the ends and create a new lipstick from the resulting mixture.

Materials for packaging were scarce too. Metal, plastic and even cardboard were needed for the war effort. Yardley got around the problem by packaging goods in wax containers. Most cosmetics came in utility packaging. Coty's Airspun Powder for example, which had once been cased in glamorous Lalique packaging, was sold in a buff coloured container inscribed 'special war pack [...] identical quality and quantity as original box'.

LATE 1940S MAKE-UP LOOK

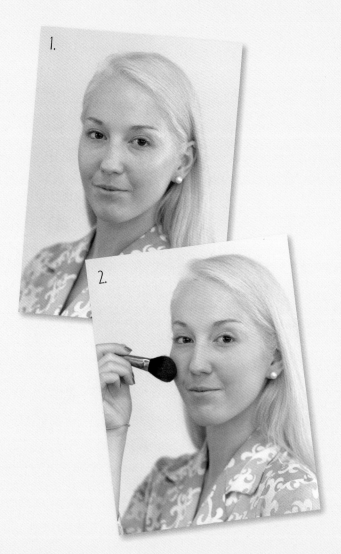

Post-war, the change in cosmetics was relatively slow. The biggest change was in eye make-up. This guide will help you to create a late decade make-up look (c.1949) like the one on p.26.

FOUNDATION

Similar to the early 1940s look, keep your foundation simple – a natural tanned colour with a dusting of powder is perfect (fig. 1).

BLUSHER

Rouge tended to be a minimal dab to emphasise a perfect bone structure (fig. 2).

BROWS

Eyebrows were perfectly shaped with a sharp eyebrow pencil. The eyebrow was slightly heavier than during wartime, although it followed relatively similar lines (fig. 3).

EYES

By the late 1940s soft doe eyes had become the most popular look, suitable for day or evening. These new eyes were created using a heavier coat of mascara and were sometimes defined with a flash of eyeliner across the upper eyelid drawn out in an elegant, dramatic flick.

More coloured eyeshadows were used in the late 40s, especially blues, greys and greens - as seen here they helped to create a more dramatic eye (fig. 3).

LIPS

Red continued to be the favoured colour for many women. There was a huge selection of red lipsticks available and also a greater variety of lighter shades including more pink and coral tones. An advertisement for Gala in 1948 offered the following shades for example: Cock's Comb; Red Bunting; Ballet Pink; Red Sequin; Heart Red; Lantern Red; Cyclamen; Heavenly Pink; Blaze; Chestnut.

Whilst increasing attention was paid to the eyes over the lips in the late 1940s, lips were still full and lipstick-coated (fig. 4).

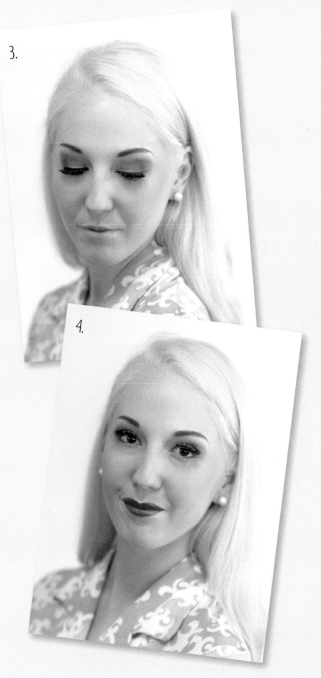

3.

4.

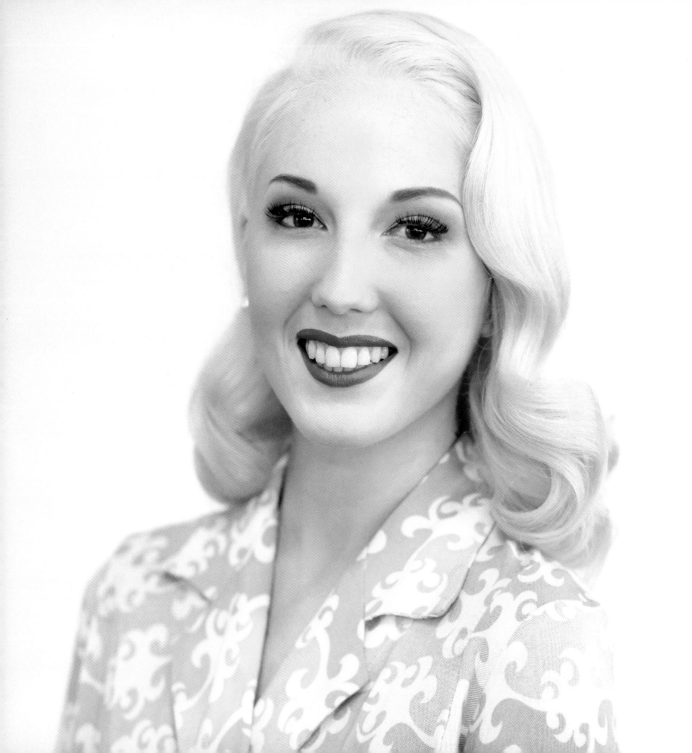

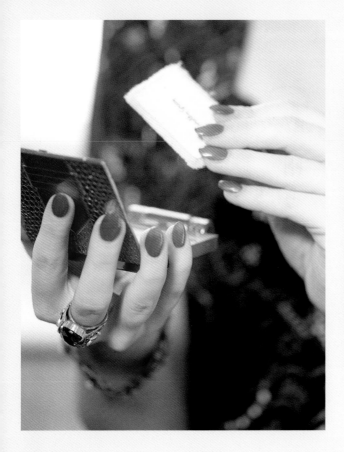

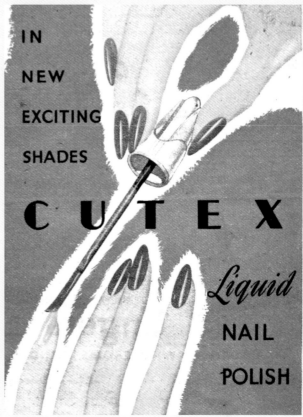

NAILS

During the early 40s many women in Europe found it difficult to acquire liquid nail polish. Therefore most simply ensured their nails were neatly manicured. For those working in factories or the services this meant keeping their nails relatively short.

If women could acquire nail polish they would paint nails to match lips. Nail colours were mainly in shades of red and pink, including darker reds and corals. Other colours were available such as gold, dark green and even black, but reds and pinks were by far the most common.

Post war, nails were long and elegant, manicured with an oval tip. Most women used either bold red or pink polish, as seen above.

Above: Advertisement for Cutex nail polish, 1948.

Hair

'I will have one of the cleanest obits of any actress. I never did cheesecake like Ann Sheridan or Betty Grable. I just used my hair.'

Veronica Lake

Despite shortages of styling products and hair accessories, the 1940s was a decade of elaborate looking hairstyles. There were a huge variety of popular styles from the pompadour to the poodle, the victory roll to the omelette fold.

For the majority of the decade, women's hair was worn in soft, feminine curls and was generally dressed off the face. The most common style was rolls of curls in decreasing sizes from a centre parting, with the back hair pinned up or left to turn under.

Warner Brothers Studios hairstylist Ivan Anderson created the 'Middy' to accommodate the intricate hairstyles and curled sets of the decade. Hair was cut in many layers, in a rounded U-shape at the back, curving up towards the ears.

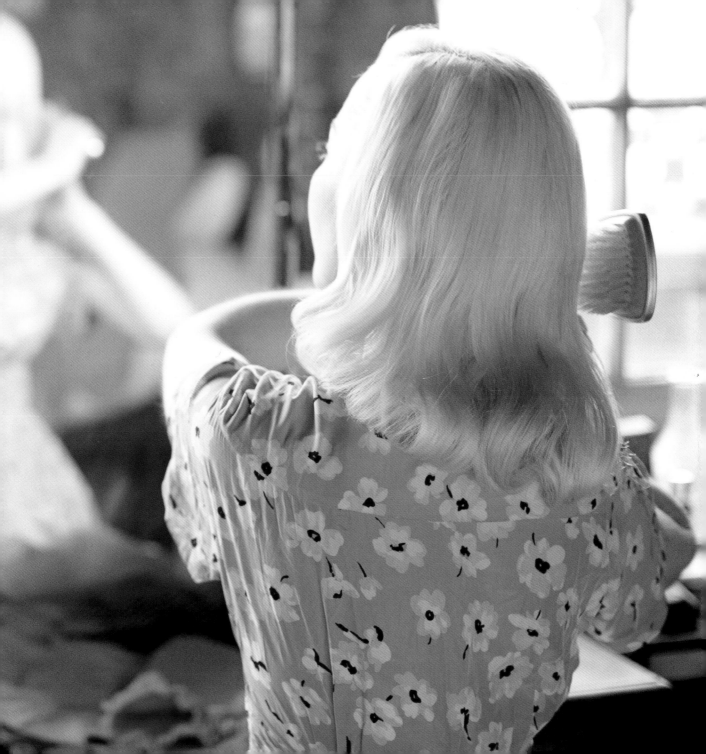

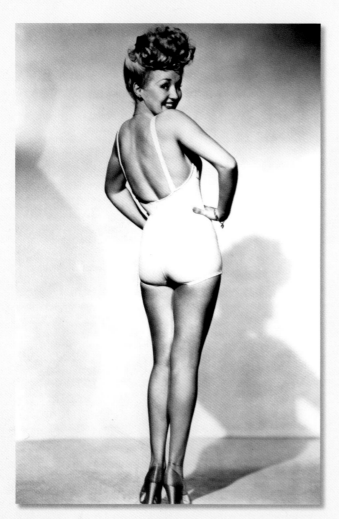

HISTORY

Hairdressing during the war was not an easy affair and by 1942 even shampoo had joined the list of hard-to-get products. Many women were limited to shampooing hair once every other week or using alternatives such as vinegar for dark hair or strained lemon for blonde. Setting lotion was also hard to come by, and both beer and sugar water were common alternatives, with pipe cleaners, rags or pin curls used to create the waves.

In the early 1940s luscious long blonde locks draped seductively over one eye were the height of hair fashion. American film star Veronica Lake promoted this style. Women ached for the glamour of Lake's look, but during wartime long hair was impractical. Some women did choose to keep their hair long, but those working in factories or in the services had to wear it rolled up under hats, turbans or snoods to ensure it was out of the way. For servicewomen the rule was that their hair could not touch the back of their collar. This meant it either had to be tightly pinned up, or cut short. In Britain short hair was far more popular, generally worn just below shoulder length or shorter.

Above: For me the film star Betty Grable epitomises 1940s hair – whether she wore her hair poodle-style, in victory rolls, or simply gently curled, she always looked effortlessly elegant.

Opposite: Veronica Lake's infamous blonde locks, 1942.

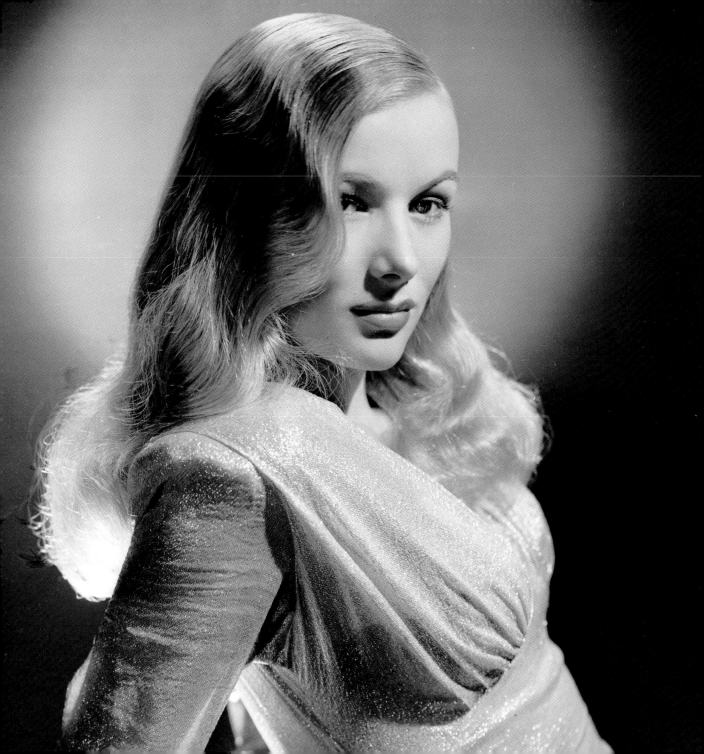

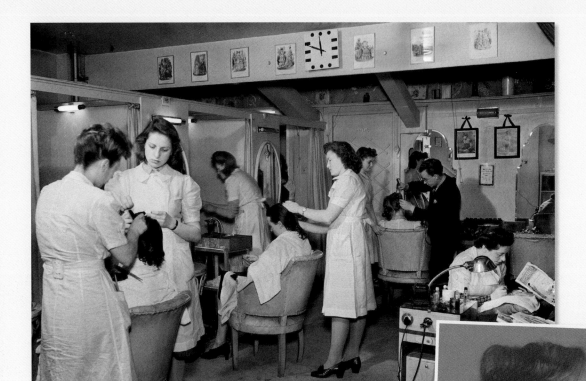

Above: Steiner's hair salon in Grosvenor Street, London (1944). The salon was housed in a basement once used as an air raid shelter.

Right: My Great Aunt Rita in 1946, with a classic mid 40s hairstyle.

Opposite: During the war even hairpins were a luxury to be hoarded, as the metal used to produce them was needed for the war effort. Women certainly did still use both grips and slides, useful for holding waves in shape and keeping hair off the face. Combs and slides made from Bakelite or faux tortoiseshell had been popular in the 30s and continued to be worn by women in the 40s.

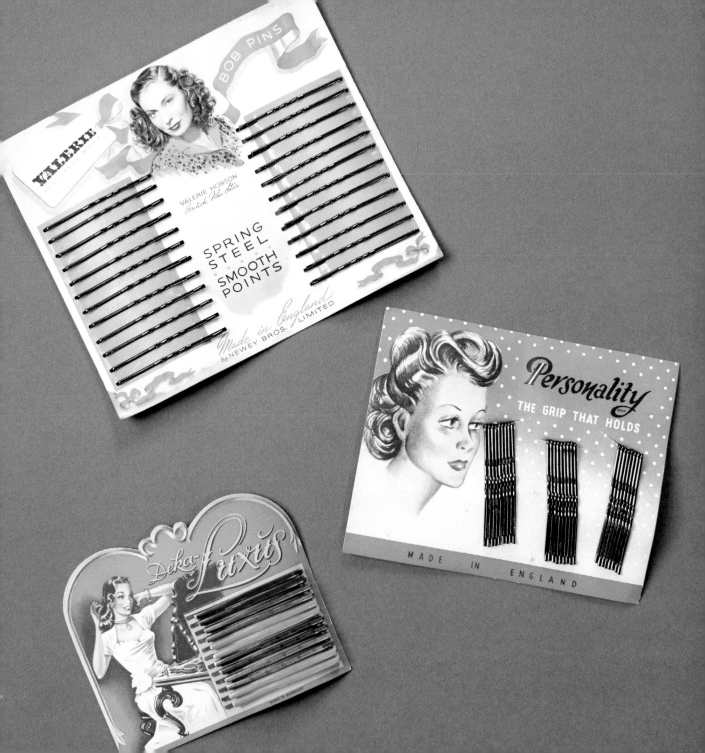

RECREATING 40S HAIRSTYLES

Here I will show you how to create a number of classic 40s hairstyles. These hairstyles are simple and can easily be done yourself. I've tried them all out myself just to make sure!

ROLLS

Rolls are a quintessential part of the 1940s look and are a flexible element of a hairstyle which can be shaped and positioned however you desire. Victory rolls are one of the most recognisable 1940s styles, popular during the decade with filmstars and ordinary women alike. The term 'victory roll' refers simply to the roll at the front of the hair, whilst the rest of the hair can be styled in a variety of manners. I believe it's best to keep it nice and simple as far as victory rolls go. Don't let them get too big if you are trying to create an accurate period look.

In the 1940s, victory rolls were often paired with soft pin curl waves. They look equally effective teamed with a pageboy style – a smooth roll going all round the back of the head and curled under. Or they could be worn simply with the rest of the hair left loose.

There are many contradicting suggestions as to where the name 'victory roll' comes from. I believe it refers to the manoeuvres completed by pilots who, on returning from battle and having successfully shot down an enemy plane, did a 'victory roll' in their plane, corkscrewing through the air before landing.

Although victory rolls are perceived as glamorous, they are quick to do and served a practical purpose, ensuring that hair was swept off the face whilst still retaining a very feminine appearance.

What you'll need

- Hairspray
- Kirby grips
- Sectioning clips
- Curling tongs
- A good quality bristle hairbrush
- A fine comb

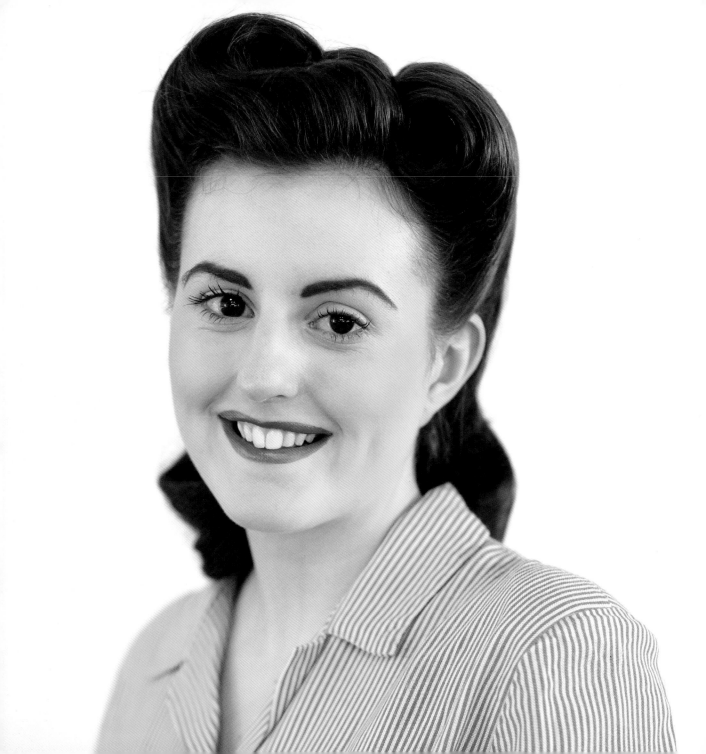

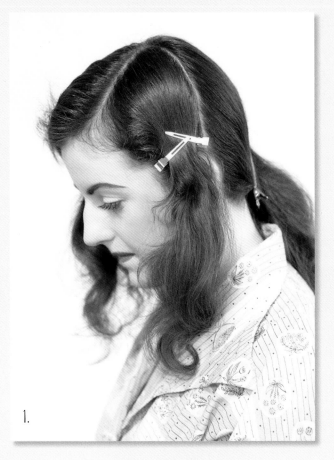

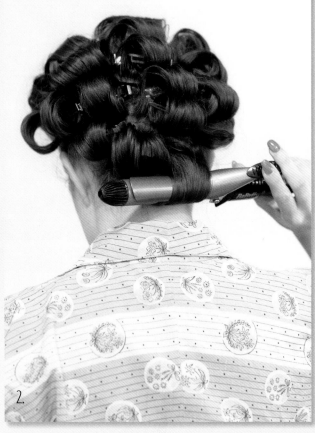

1. Part the hair low on one side. Section hair from the crown to behind the ears on both sides and clip with control grips. This will leave you with three sections of hair [fig. 1].

2. Curl small sections of hair with tongs and clip into place. Curl the front sections to the side and the back section under [fig. 2].

TOP TIP
For extra hold apply setting lotion to the hair before you begin this style.

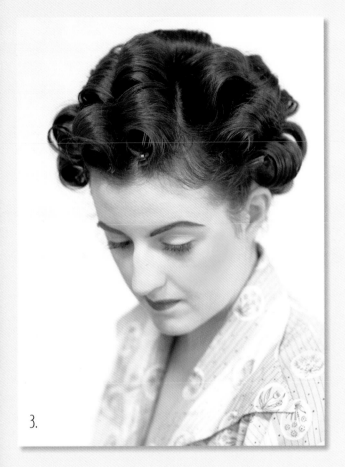

3.

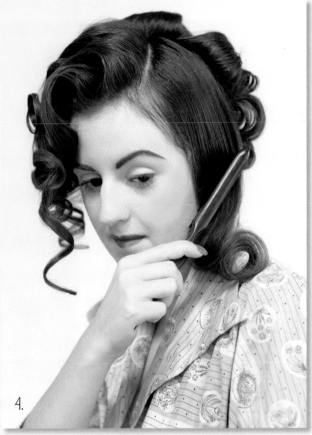

4.

3. Leave until the hair is fully cooled, or dry if using setting lotion [fig. 3].

4. Begin to take out the curls in the side sections and brush through. The curls should retain some bounce [fig. 4].

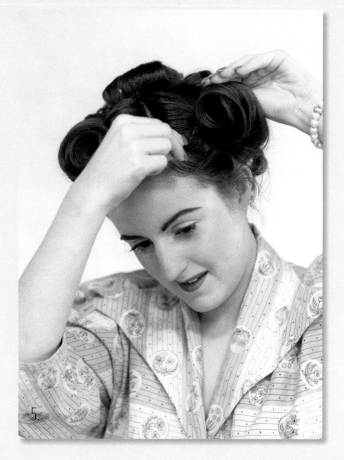

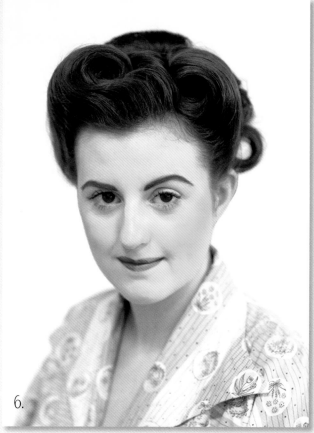

5. Curl each side section around your hand into a roll, curling upwards towards the parting, and pin into place at the base of the curl. Try to put the grip right inside the roll so it will not show when the style is finished. Smooth stray strands into the rolls and apply hairspray to fix [fig. 5].

6. The finished effect shoud look like this at the front [fig. 6].

7. Finally, take the curls out of the back section and brush through, curling the ends under. Spritz with a little hairspray to hold the style in place [fig. 7].

TOP TIP

If your hair is particularly fine backcomb each section before you roll it.

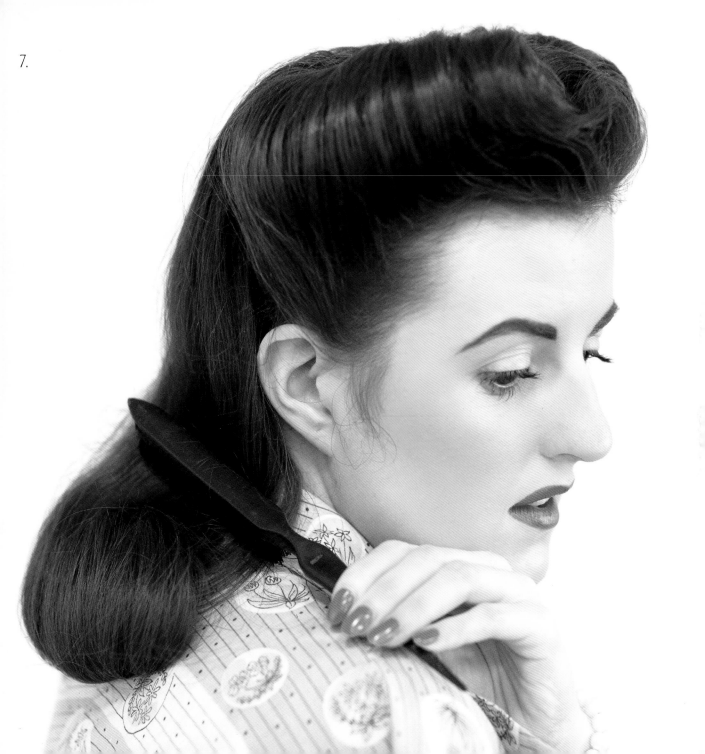

7.

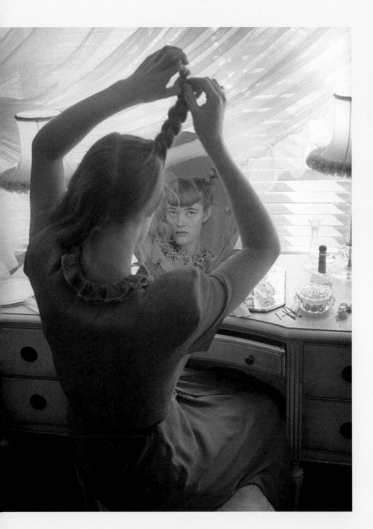

Above: A young girl braiding her hair in 1948.

BRAIDS

Braids were fashionable throughout the decade. Women with long hair could braid their own on top of their head, or those with shorter hair could add hairpieces. This style was particularly popular in America, and was often seen in the beauty pages of American *Vogue*. Hairpieces in contrasting colours were sometimes used. A piece of material or a long thin scarf plaited with the hair made a colourful alternative. Braids could be worn on various points of the head, although most often coiled around the crown or on top of the head like a hairband.

What you'll need
- Hairspray
- Hair grips
- Sectioning clips
- Hair elastic
- Hairbrush

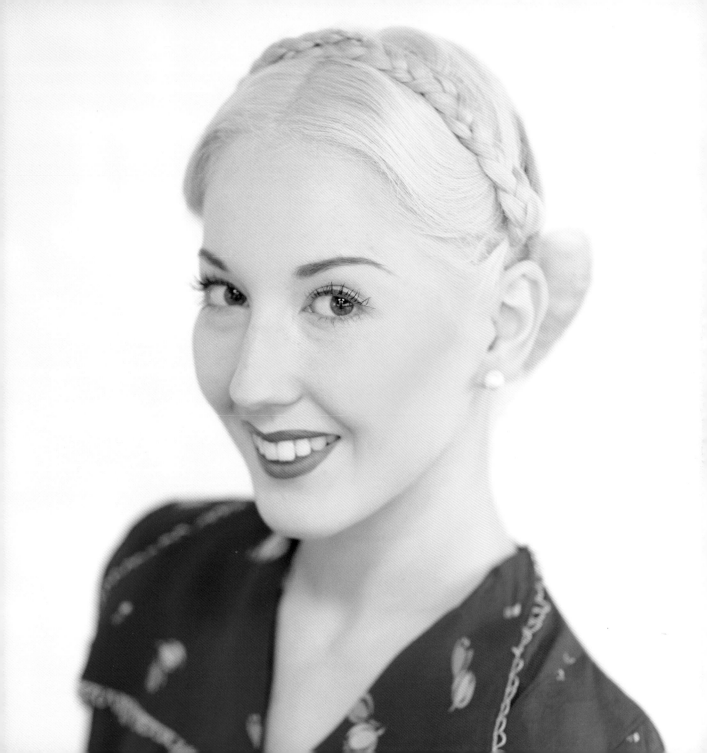

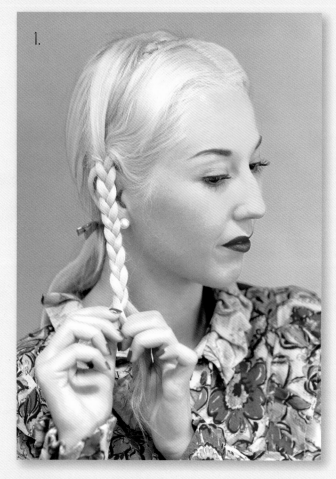

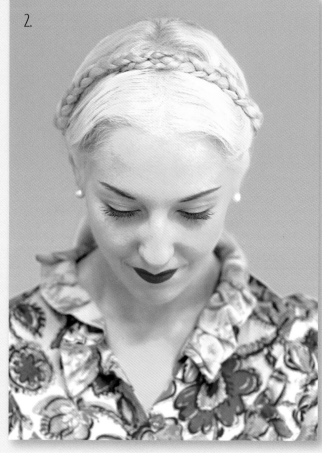

This style works best with a middle parting and shoulder length or longer hair.

1. Section hair from the crown to behind the ears on both sides and clip the remainder of the hair into a loose ponytail at the nape of your neck. Create a skinny plait with the front section of your hair on both sides. Secure with a clear hair elastic (fig. 1).

2. Cross the plaits over the top of your head and secure the ends of the plaits underneath each other with a hairpin so that it looks like one continuous plait.

3. Tie up the back of the hair into a standard ponytail. Secure with a hair elastic. Wrap a single piece of hair over the hair elastic to cover it and secure with a hair grip.

3.

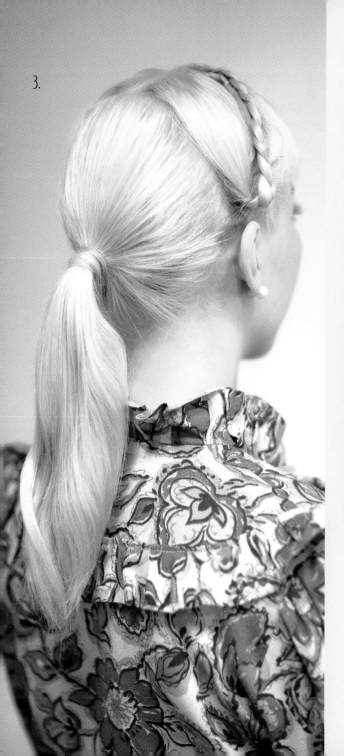

4.

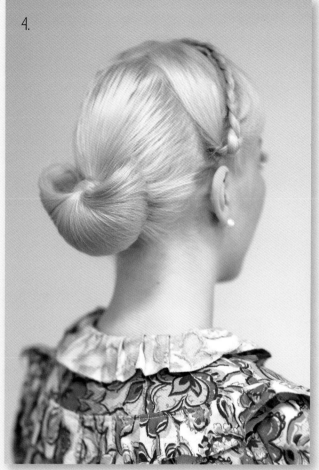

4. To create the fan shape- curl the hair under in a roll and gentle fan it out both sides. Secure the sides with grips.

5. To finish off the style spritz with a little hairspray.

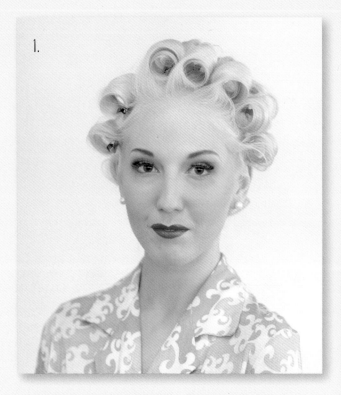

1.

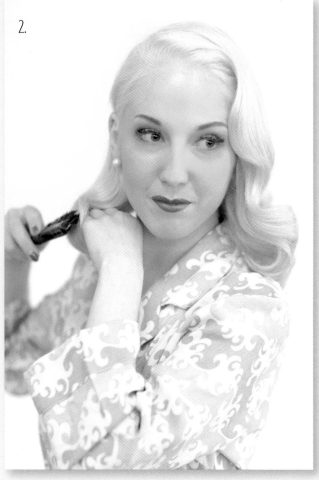

2.

HOLLYWOOD WAVES

This style works best with long hair.

1. Part the hair low on one side. Curl the hair with tongs starting from the parting. Ensure all the curls are rolled under as this will mean the waves go in the correct direction. Pin each curl in place with a sectioning grip and leave the hair to cool down.

2. Remove clips and brush out the hair gently. Spritz with hairspray to hold the style in place.

What you'll need
- Curling tongs
- Sectioning clips
- Hairspray
- Hairbrush

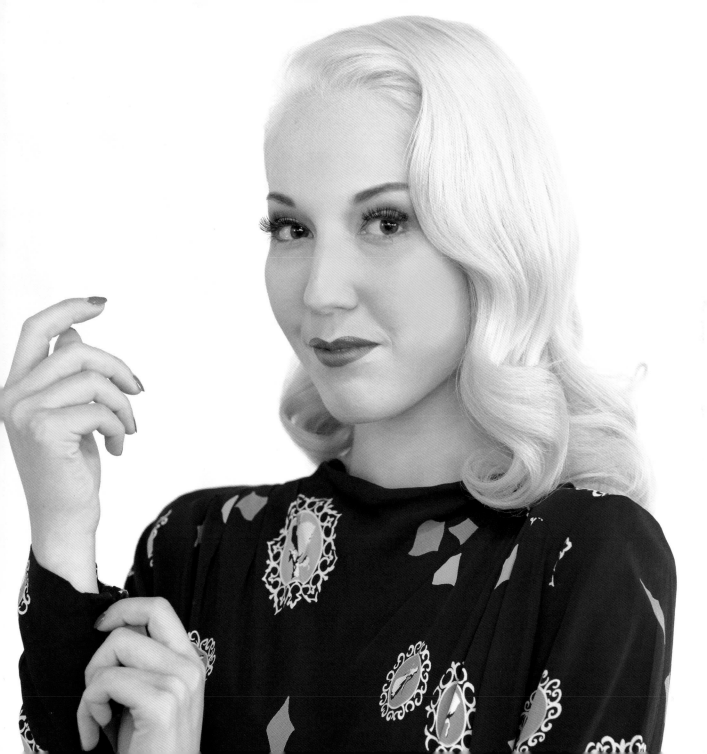

HEAD COVERINGS

For factory and farm work it was necessary for women to keep long hair covered up and away from dangerous machinery. Many women wore their hair in pin curls beneath turbans and headscarves. This meant hair could easily be let down, spruced up and dressed up after work. Head coverings such as turbans and scarves also served the practical purpose of covering unwashed hair.

TURBANS AND HEADSCARVES

Turbans were generally made from a length of soft material such as a fine wool or rayon crepe. The fabric was tied on top of the head and the long ends were then simply tucked under, or rolled up first then tucked under, to create a more defined U-shape. The turban could be left as it was or decorated with things like flowers for a more dressy look. Women in the 1940s often referred to headscarves as turbans too.

During the 1940s scarves came in a variety of materials, sizes and patterns and were worn in numerous ways. They could be plaited into the hair and tied up, folded into a triangle and tied on top of the head, or simply worn around the head and knotted under the chin. See overleaf for a scarf tying tutorial.

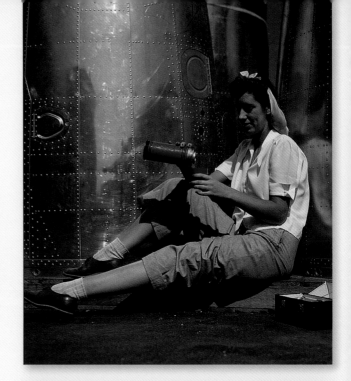

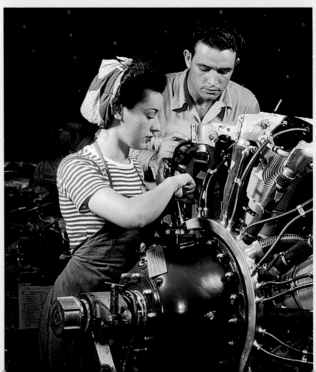

Right: Female employees of the Californian Douglas Aircraft company in 1942, wearing a snood (top) and a headscarf (bottom).

SNOODS

The snood was a net, worn alone or with a hat, that contained the hair at the back of the head. It had been popular in the nineteenth century and was re-introduced by Schiaparelli in 1935. However it really only came into general use at the advent of war, as a means of keeping hair covered. In some factories snoods were supplied along with other protective clothing, to keep hair away from machinery.

HATS

Whilst social trends had previously dictated that hats were a necessity, during the war they were seen as a frivolity. Women still wore hats but largely for formal occasions only. Whilst hats were not rationed they were prohibitively expensive and few women could afford to buy new. Women were still making smaller hats and headpieces from oddments of material that they could find – felt, straw and ribbons for example – or refashioning old hats into new.

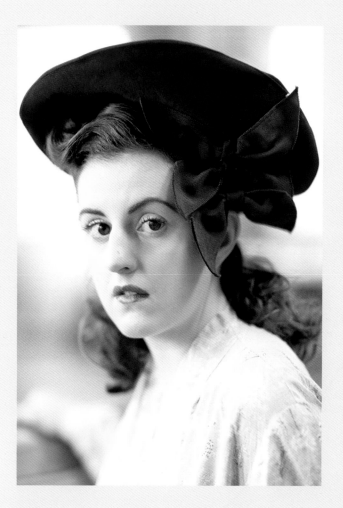

Above: Holly wears a navy blue felt tilted pancake hat with statement bow details.

'Before the war, to go out without a hat was to go out half dressed.'
Vogue, August 1942

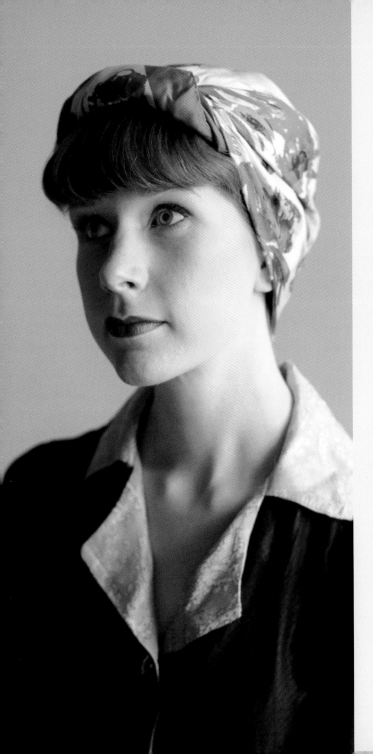

HOW TO TIE THE PERFECT 40S HEADSCARF

In my opinion it's best to use a large square scarf for this style, but it can also work with a triangular scarf left unfolded.

1. Fold the scarf in half.

2. Pull the scarf around your head. The long straight end should go to the back of your head and sit around the nape of your neck [fig. 1].

3. Rearrange so that the points rest roughly at eye level.

4. Take both of the long hanging ends and pull them to the top of your head.

5. Twist them together in a knot [fig. 2], you should now have two hanging 'bunny's ears' and a point at the front of your forehead.

6. Tuck the bunny's ears in the two holes that should have developed at the side of the scarf [fig. 3].

7. Roll and tuck the hanging point over the knot [fig. 4].

8. Pop a hairgrip in at either side to hold the headscarf in place.

9. Et Voilà! The perfect 40s headscarf.

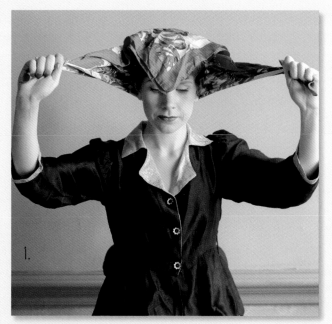

1.

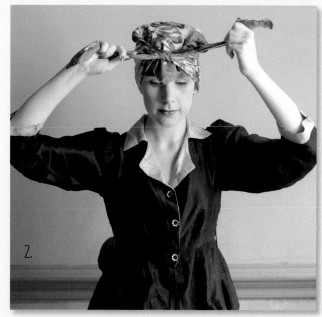

2.

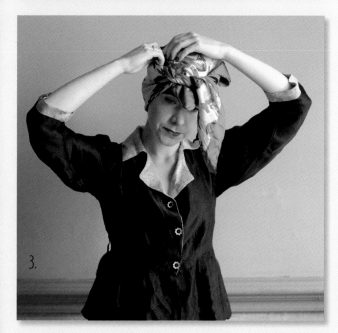

3.

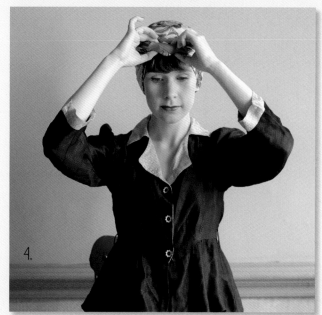

4.

Wartime Fashion

'Mend and Make-do to save buying new.'

British WWII propaganda slogan

During World War II, British women had to cope with restrictions upon their wardrobes. War resulted in a shortage of labour and materials and therefore constraints were imposed upon manufacturers and consumers alike. How a woman dressed was no longer dictated by her taste or wealth but by wartime conditions and controls set down by the government.

Similarly in other parts of Europe women faced extreme restrictions upon their wardrobes. Women in occupied Paris turned to their own creativity to ensure they still looked chic, whilst in Germany it was incredibly difficult to acquire even the most basic clothes.

America on the other hand was able to build its fashion industry from strength to strength. Cut off from Europe by war a truly American style was beginning to develop and would soon be influencing fashion styles around the world.

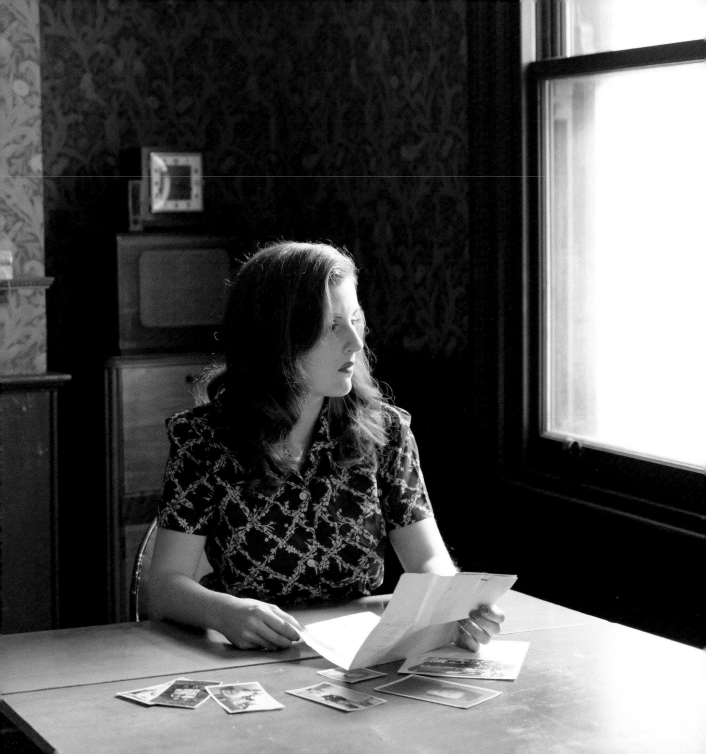

FASHION ON THE RATION

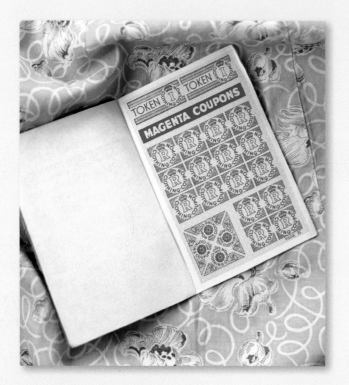

In Britain during the war, simplicity was the key word. Dresses were manufactured without fancy trims and stitching, whilst seams and buttons served only functional purposes as opposed to decorative. Metal was desperately needed for the war effort, meaning fewer garments had metal zips – most manufacturers resorted to fastenings of either poppers or buttons. Garments were designed to be hard-wearing and sensible – like the morale of the British people, they were built to stand the test of war.

Above: An original late 1940s ration book.

'Fashion, like the woman it clothes, is proving no good-time girl, thrown into confusion by the shock of war, but a staunch support, an invaluable ally.' Vogue, November 1939

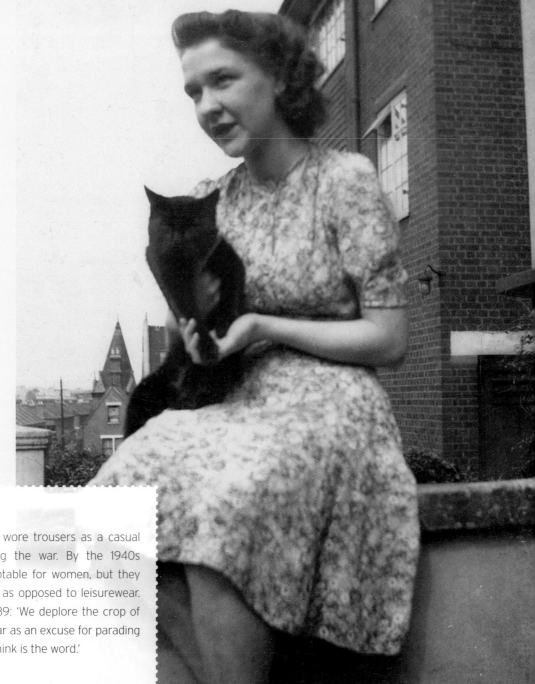

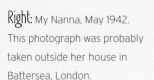 My Nanna, May 1942. This photograph was probably taken outside her house in Battersea, London.

Slacks: The wartime myth

Very few women actually wore trousers as a casual garment in Britain during the war. By the 1940s trousers were more acceptable for women, but they were viewed as workwear as opposed to leisurewear. *British Vogue* stated in 1939: 'We deplore the crop of young women who take war as an excuse for parading about in slacks. Slack we think is the word.'

RATIONING

Between 1939 and 1941 the general cost of living in Britain soared by 29%, but the price of clothing had grown even faster, increasing by 69%. These price increases left many people unable to buy even the most essential garments. The government recognised that the cost of clothing had to be stabilised, and rationing was the fairest way to go about it. Rationing was designed to reduce consumer spending, free up valuable factory space and release workers for the war industries.

Clothes rationing was introduced in June 1941. Initially there were no clothes ration books – consumers used special 'margarine' coupons in the back of their food ration books to purchase clothing. This was a clever tactic on behalf of the government. They feared that if hundreds of thousands of clothes ration books were printed it would incite panic buying in consumers. The coupon system meant that both cash and coupons were required for the purchase of clothing.

DID YOU KNOW?

The British rationing system was based on the German rationing plan of 1939 with additions and amendments thought up by government scientists in co-operation with technologists from Marks and Spencer.

In 1941 each adult was allowed 66 coupons for the purchase of clothes per year. By 1943, owing to shortages, this was reduced to 48. The coupon system was confusing and until rationing ended in 1949 the number of coupons allocated each year yo-yoed. Post-war, coupon numbers rose again and there were roughly 67 coupons per person in 1947.

This may seem very restrictive, but there were certainly ways of getting around rationing and acquiring clothes. Second-hand clothing was not rationed as it presented administrative problems. Furthermore, it wasn't uncommon for elderly people to offer coupons to grandchildren or younger relatives. There was also a thriving black market both in coupons and supposed 'second-hand' clothes which sometimes transpired to be stolen new goods. My Nanna acquired extra coupons from her sister who worked as a cashier. Completely illegal, but if you were a fashionable young woman as my Nanna was, you would do anything for new clothes!

In February 1942 the Utility scheme was introduced to try to curb the still rising prices of clothes. Rationing imposed restrictions on consumer purchasing. Utility on the other hand imposed restrictions on the manufacturer. The Utility scheme helped to control both the price and quality of clothing and all Utility garments carried a 'CC41' label (see page 58). In 1942 50% of all clothing produced came under Utility, but by 1945 this had increased to 85%, demonstrating how popular the scheme was with manufacturers.

Coupon values for women

- Lined coat over 71cm in length: 14
- Jacket or short coat: 11
- Wool dress: 11
- Non-wool dress: 7
- Blouse, cardigan or jumper: 5
- Skirt or culottes: 7
- Shoes, boots or slippers: 5
- Stockings: 2
- Slip, petticoat, cami-knickers or combination garment: 4
- Corset or other underwear: 3
- Ankle socks: 1
- Pyjamas: 8
- Nightdress: 6
- Overalls or dungarees: 6
- Apron: 3
- Collar, tie or pair of cuffs: 1
- Two handkerchiefs: 1
- Scarf, pair of gloves, mittens or muff: 2

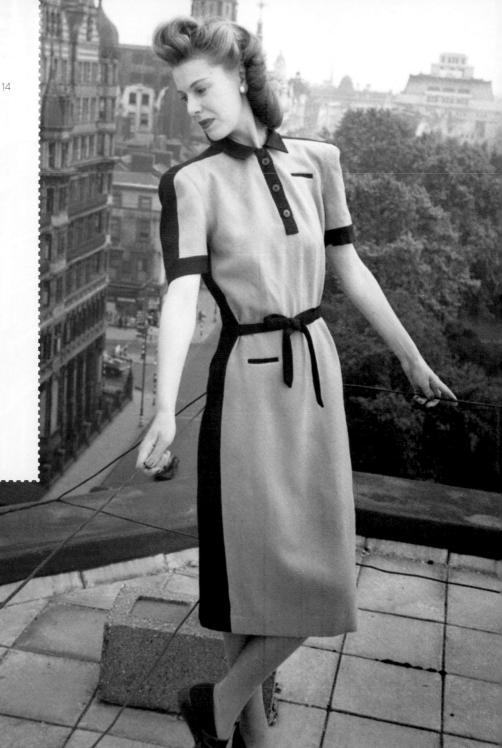

Right: A pale blue and black wool Utility dress by British brand Atrima (Rima), 1943. The dress required 11 coupons.

Owing to the restrictions imposed on manufacturers Utility clothes were the best quality available. Dresses for example were made of rayon that wouldn't shrink and dyes that wouldn't run or bleed. However, there were complaints about Utility clothing. Most of these came from consumers who were used to purchasing luxury garments and viewed Utility as substandard.

Whilst not all firms participated in the Utility scheme ALL (even those creating bespoke designs) were supposed to adhere to austerity measures or the 'Making of Civilian Clothing (Restrictions) Orders'. These orders were passed in 1942 and 1943 and aimed to remove all non-essential elements (such as trims and embroideries) from garments thus saving time and money in the manufacturing process. Even fabric designs were influenced by austerity measures, as dainty floral and figurative patterns were easier to match up and hence created less wastage in production. The austerity rulings were exhaustive. There were at least 18 restrictions on skirts alone. Here are just a few restrictions that applied to women's dresses.

Dresses could not have:

- more than 2 pockets
- embroidery (hand or machine), applique, applique work, applique embroidery, braid, quilting (including puffing and matelasse), beading, sequins, rouleaux work (except for one row as a finish for the neck or sleeves), drawn thread work, galloons, or lace or lace-net trimmings
- tiered skirts
- capes
- turn-back cuffs
- imitation pockets
- buttons for the purposes of ornament
- Depth of hem over 2"

Seemingly not all manufacturers adhered to the restrictions as examples can be found that don't fit within these remits. In 1944 some of these restrictions were removed which may be why so many examples of mid-40s garments are found with restricted features (beading and sequins, I'm looking at you!).

NON-RATIONED GOODS

Most clothing was rationed, but a few items escaped rationing:

- Heavily taxed luxury items (fur coats, lace and hats)
- All sewing threads, braids and ribbons under 3in
- Boiler suits
- Sanitary towels
- Clogs
- Braces
- Garters
- Boot/shoelaces

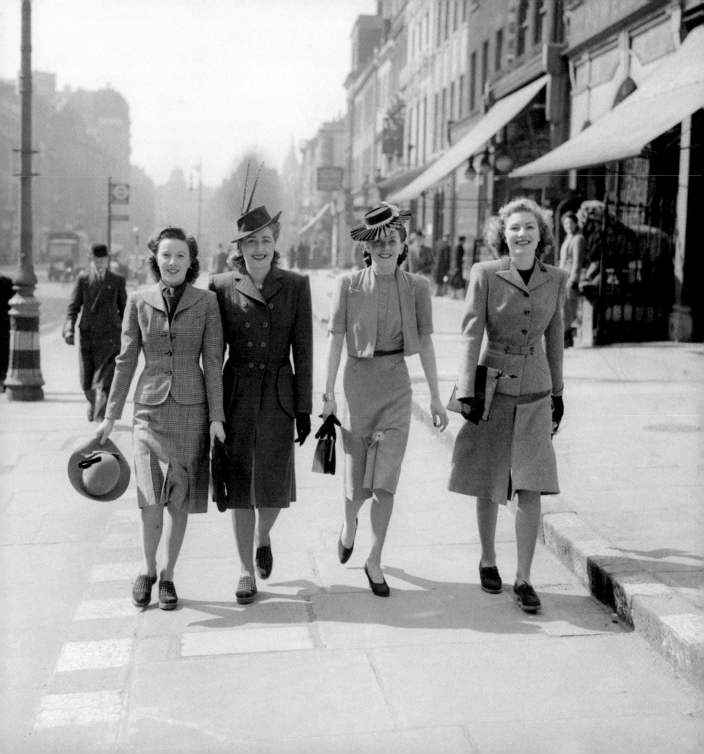

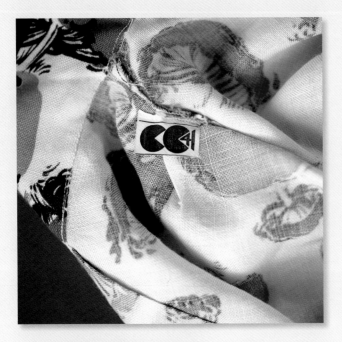

Left: The stylised double c, label, denotes a standard Utility product. Reginald Shipp, a commercial designer for Hargreaves, designed this label.

Bottom left: The high street store Marks and Spencer is often associated with Utility. The company worked on tiny profit margins meaning it could offer garments at lower prices than those set by the Board of Trade. They were one of the few companies to retain their brand label in their products (many disappeared in 1942).

Opposite: Two Utility dresses designed by British couturier Norman Hartnell for Berketex, 1942. On the left is a navy blue wool dress. The yoke is scarlet with pale blue inserts. On the right a long sleeve dress in red and black Scotch tweed.

Below: The double elevens or 'dinner plate' label denotes a luxury Utility product. It is thought this label was introduced post-1945 due to the negative connotations associated with the double c logo.

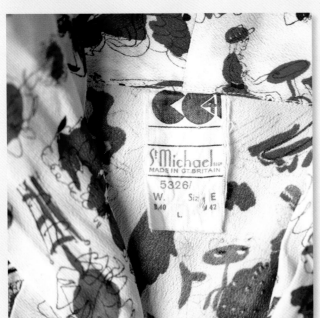

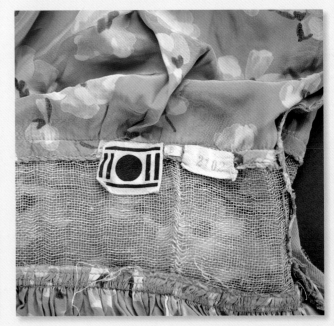

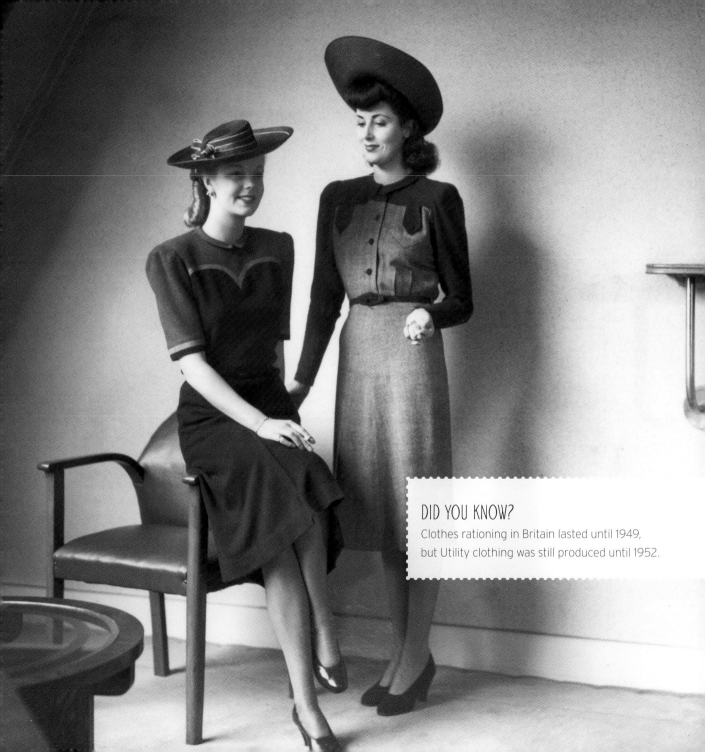

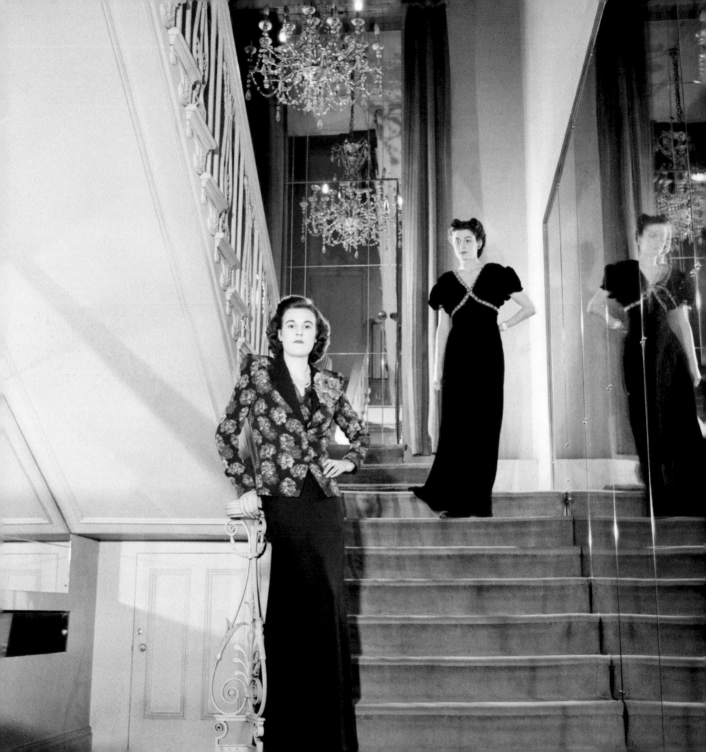

INCSOC

Whilst British fashion is not often celebrated for its couturiers during the Second World War, British couture created hugely important overseas income to support the war effort.

In 1942 the Incorporated Society of London Fashion Designers was established. This organisation represented the crème de la crème of British couturiers and included names such as Norman Hartnell, Hardy Amies and Digby Morton. IncSoc aimed to promote the British fashion and textile industry at home and abroad.

During the spring of 1942 the Board of Trade asked IncSoc members to create a series of designs using Utility fabrics and conforming to austerity rulings. The couturiers' designs were shown in a September 1942 fashion show. The models were all war workers who had volunteered their time. Individual couturiers were not credited for these designs, but they became prototypes for garments produced by the ready-to-wear sector of the British fashion industry.

Left: Two models pose on the staircase of Norman Hartnell's fashion house (Hartnell was a founder member of IncSoc). The model at the top of stairs wears a black velvet dinner gown studded in blue and gold. In the foreground, the model wears a crêpe dinner suit.

FABRICS

Many commonly used clothing fabrics were in short supply during the war. By 1941 the shortage of silk, leather and wool was dire. Home dressmakers and companies alike began to look for alternatives. Rayon became one of the most popular fabrics of the decade as it was both practical and economical. Heavy linen-esque rayon was used for suits, whilst lighter crêpe rayon was used for dresses and blouses. Rayon was also utilised to create jersey, faille and taffeta. Other fashionable wartime fabrics included velvet, velveteen, moygashel and corduroy.

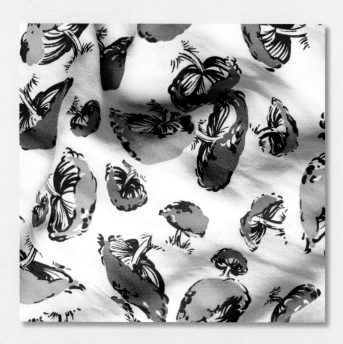

COLOURS

Often wartime fashion is associated with dull and drab colours, but I think this paints an inaccurate picture. Black and white film footage and photographs only emphasise the feeling of the dull drabness of war. Yet women were certainly wearing bright exciting garments, as some of my favourite wartime pieces shown here demonstrate.

Early on in the war colours were largely understated – blues, browns, greens and blacks. Clothing companies and magazines advertised patriotic names for garment colours – Air Force Blue, Flag Red and Army Tan for example. But in 1942, as *Homes and Gardens* magazine suggested, vibrant colours were already being combined for interesting effect – 'there are brown frocks with tomato fronts, pale blue fronts, or gold brocade fronts, black with cherry or emerald.' *Vogue* also stated that firms were using colour in bold ways. It celebrated that summer 1944 was the season of two colour prints: 'Crisp white on black, or navy on red in geometric prints [...] Squares, stripes and dots and small clear motifs.'

Left: A mushroom print moygashel summer dress featuring a standard cc41 label , c.1945.

Opposite: A novelty print rayon dress by St. Michael featuring a standard cc41 label , c.1943.

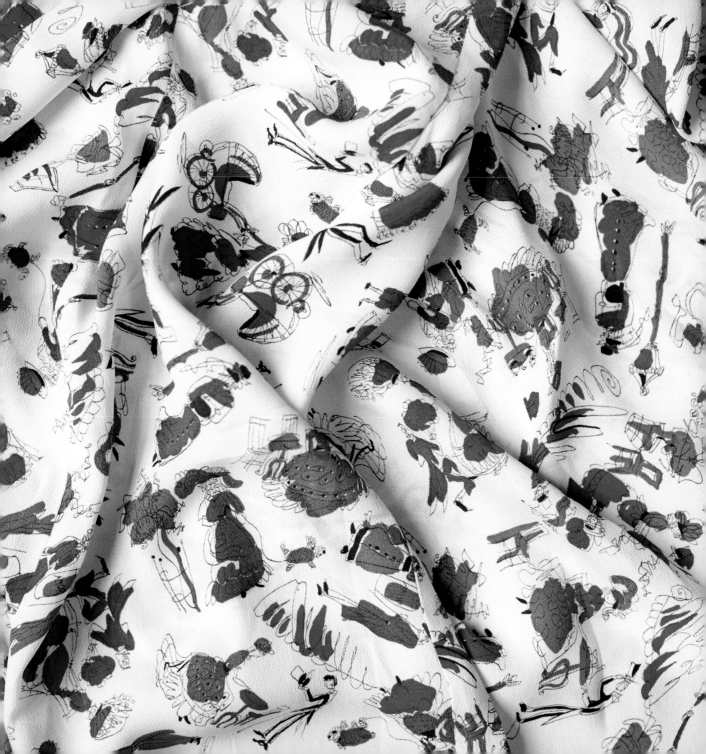

DAYTIME LOOK

Here are a few features that define a 1940s British daytime look. Such a look can easily be recreated with modern clothes.

SUIT

A good matching suit will always be a great base for a 40s look. Try to stay away from black suits as, owing to the large amount of dye needed, these weren't too common during the war. A simple, plain, modern wool suit with the right accessories can pass for the real deal. A modern tweed jacket teamed with a plain straight (as opposed to pencil) skirt can also recreate the look effectively.

Suits should be:
- Neatly tailored
- Skirts at around knee-length and straight cut
- Cut in a relatively masculine way – ideally with gently padded shoulders
- In shades of grey, dark blue, brown, or dark green
- Made from durable materials such as tweed and wool

BLOUSES
- Simple in shape with either a wide or Peter Pan collar
- Muted in colour with very small prints. These can be novelty or floral

DRESSES
- Button down and shirtwaist dresses in cotton or rayon
- Styles that can be worn from day to evening

COATS
- Masculine looking and often slightly oversized (great for fitting lots of layers underneath!)

SHOES
- Flat brogue lace-up
- Low heeled platform

Opposite: Rosy wears an elegant two-piece wool tweed suit, black felt hat and Lotus red snakeskin platform shoes. Holly wears a St. Michael powder blue coat and St. Michael novelty print dress dated c.1943. Her shoes are by Rayne.

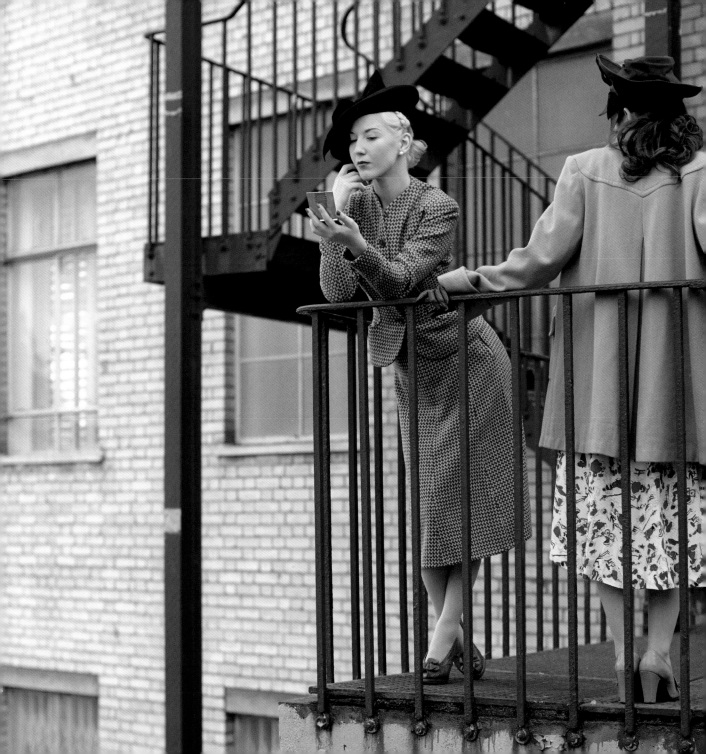

EVENING LOOK

People's social lives were seriously affected by the war and there were no longer many grand formal occasions. Early on in the war women were still wearing mid to late 30s garments for formal occasions, but by the mid 1940s these had often been converted to more useful garments. Instead, for smart occasions British women largely wore a simple evening skirt and blouse, or a day dress.

DRESSES

- 1930s adapted evening dresses
- Day dresses
- A simple skirt and blouse
- Narrow skirts
- Peg top skirts
- Deep cut armholes

SHOES

- 1930s evening shoes were still largely worn
- If they could afford it (and had the coupons!) women sometimes wore gold or silver buttersoft leather strappy shoes with small platforms and a thick, chunky heel

ACCESSORIES

- Dainty 30s handbags
- An animal skin clutch
- A fur stole to keep you warm on chilly wartime nights

Opposite: This satin evening dress was made in the late 1930s, but was altered in the 1940s to fit in with the wartime silhouette. The sleeves were made narrower and a side zip fastening was added for ease of wear.

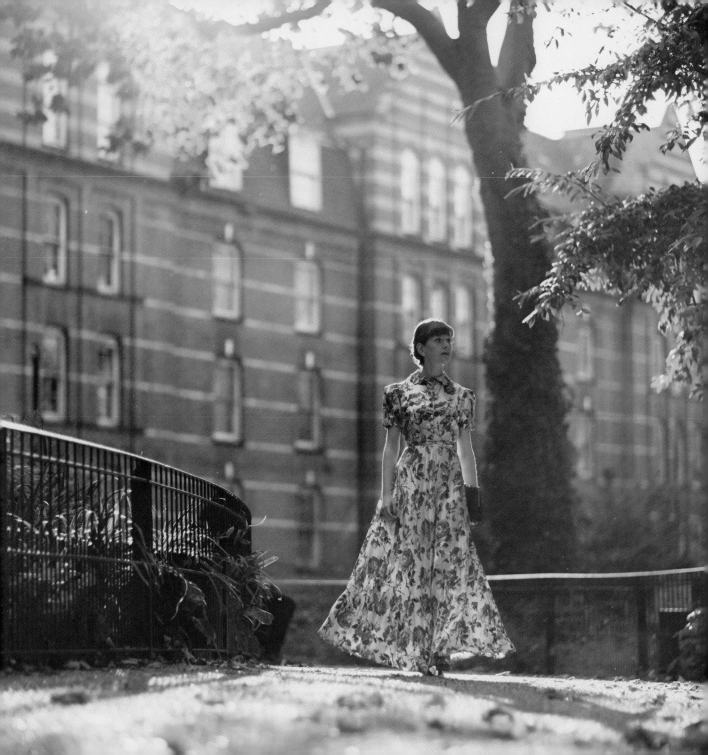

'Let's furnish our homes and wardrobes with all our economic inventiveness, using up just scraps and oddments. Let's make-over and make-out with what we've got somehow. Let's not just make do though. Old, tired wardrobes and dull, dreary rooms are admissions of defeat.' Vogue, April 1943

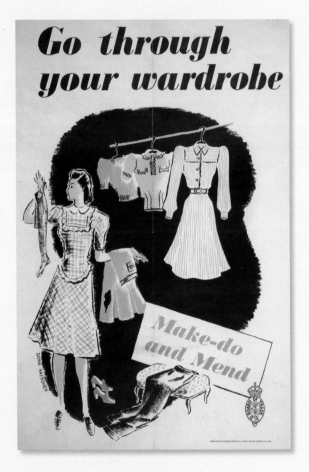

MAKE-DO AND MEND

The dearth of clothes in British shops by 1940 coupled with rapid price increases meant that people everywhere had to make do and mend. Women needed to be inventive with their clothes – they used ingenious tricks to refashion new clothing from old and thought of ways to ensure that they got the longest usage possible from garments.

For poorer sections of the nation, patching and mending old clothes and passing them down to relatives and friends had always been the way. Therefore, the Make-do and Mend campaign was largely directed towards the middle and upper classes who had no prior experience of having to do such things. Special Make-do and Mend pamphlets offered advice (you can buy re-prints of these today) and magazines offered tips too. Some even produced special issues with handy hints. British *Vogue*'s April 1943 issue for example was entitled 'spring renovations for house and wardrobe'.

Right: Holly wears a lavender crêpe day dress. It is likely this dress was originally pale blue but was dyed this shade of lavender during the war.

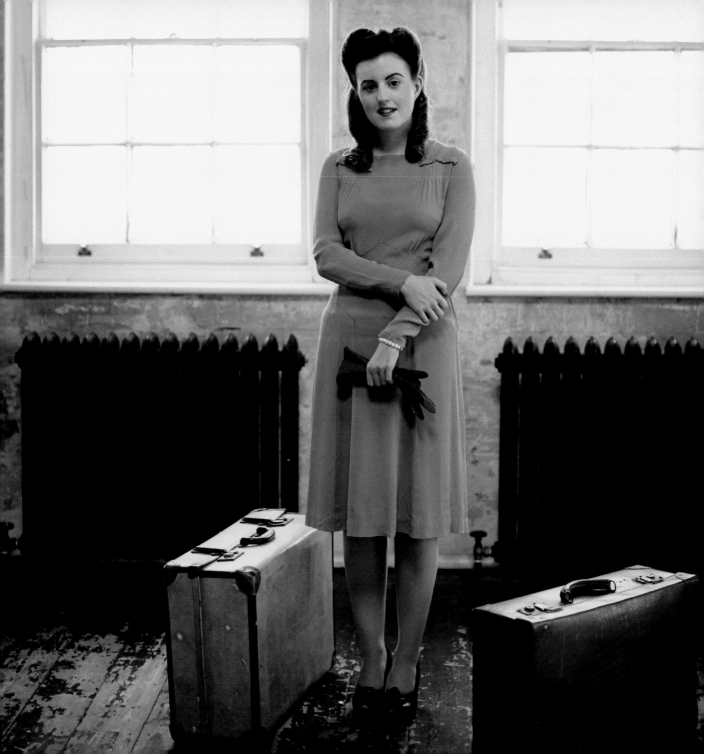

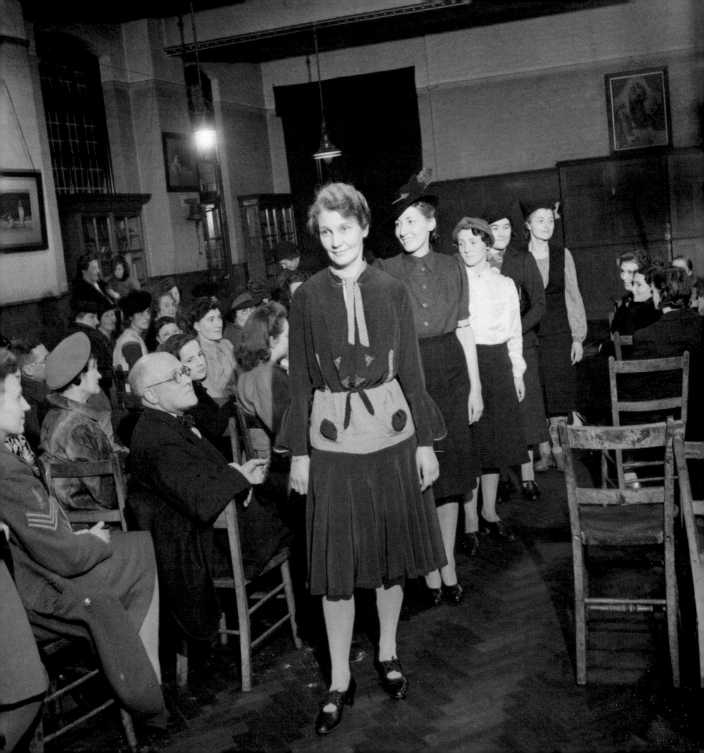

Anything and everything was creatively turned into new garments: blankets were made into coats or dressing gowns; old evening dresses turned into lingerie; furnishing fabrics used for dresses; absent men's clothes re-fashioned into women's ones. A Lux soap advert even claimed that 'the best parts of worn out lace curtains can make lovely brassieres.'

Women often customised existing pieces to ensure that they had a longer life, or were just a little more exciting. Plain garments were jazzed up with paint, embroidery and homemade trimmings. When garments became shabby problem areas such as underarms and elbows were patched with contrasting panels of fabric.

Make-do and Mend was not just an activity practised by home dressmakers. If you could afford it there were specialist services offering new clothes without coupons – old coats re-fashioned into new or simply altering dresses to new lengths and styles. Private dressmakers also offered 'reconfectioning' services – removing frills etc. from dresses and putting them to other uses. *Vogue*'s Shop Hound reported in 1943 that John Lewis and Peter Jones would undertake 'almost anything', whether mending a broken plate or making a dress out of a pair of flannel trousers. Bourne and Hollingsworth were also mentioned for remodelling dresses and hats and Leathercraft could re-fashion leather coats.

'Vogue' top tips – April 1943

- Embellish a black dress with patch pockets made from a paisley handkerchief cut in half.
- Change your shirt by fastening it with crisp ribbon bows of different colours instead of buttons.
- Refresh a dull navy blue suit with a border of coarse navy lace around cuff and collar.

DID YOU KNOW

Parachute silk was highly prized for underwear, nightclothes and wedding dresses. During the war women acquired it on the black market or from fallen parachutes. From 1945 parachutes were on open sale and could be bought from many stores.

Left: During the 1940s most women were adept seamstresses, so re-fashioning clothing would not have been too complicated. But for those who struggled special Make-do and Mend classes were set up. This image shows a class in 1943.

KNITWEAR

Despite extreme wool shortages during the war knitted garments were a staple of women's wardrobes, whether they were homemade or shop bought. Knitted garments were incredibly popular owing to their practicality and versatility. They were warm without being too heavy or restrictive and they could be washed easily.

Inventive knitters unravelled out-dated, outsized or moth-eaten items to re-use the wool. Fancy knitting techniques such as lace stitches and openwork knits made the most of limited resources and often garments were made using either a twisted rib or moss stitch as these were particularly hard wearing. Complex multi-coloured Fair Isle patterns were all the rage as they could be created with oddments of wool.

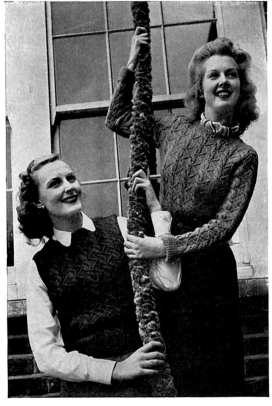

"Hallo twins!" And believe it or not, the cable pullover and the sleeveless jerkin are knitted from the same design. The pullover with sleeves is the sort of knitted that has become a real necessity for the out-of-doors girl.

Above: Two cheerful looking ladies model a cable pullover and a sleeveless jerkin, made from the same knitting pattern in "Knitting for all Illustrated" by Margaret Murray and Jane Koster, circa 1941.

Right: Holly wears a sweet European 1940s cardigan. This number was probably mass-produced.

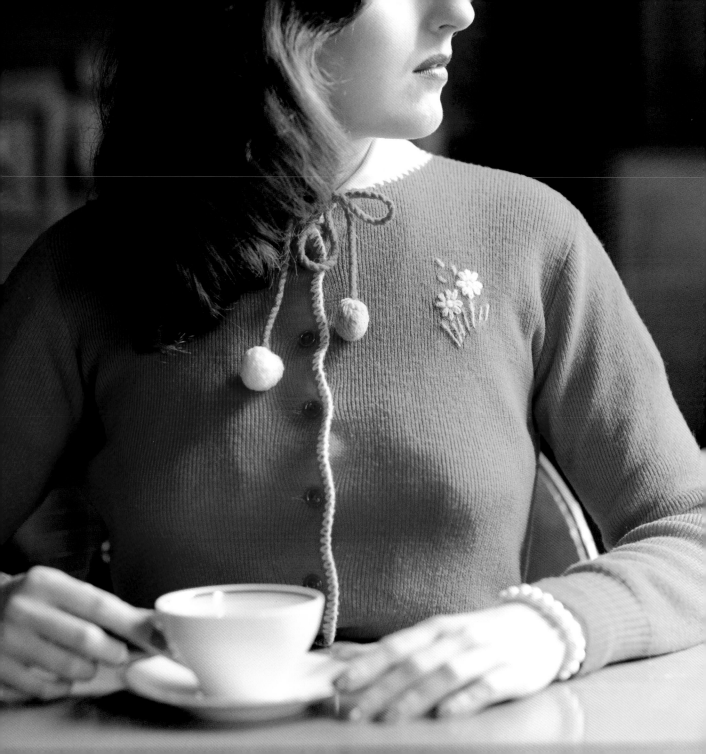

WOMEN AND WAR WORK

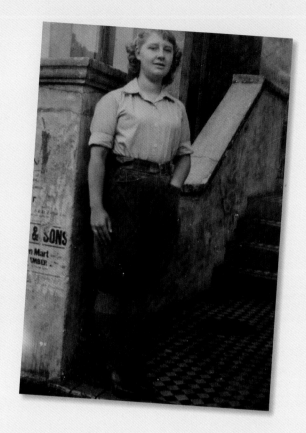

Women played a major role during WW2 and attitudes to women in the workforce were changed forever. The roles played by women had huge knock-on effects for the way women dressed – they were performing unfamiliar job roles in unfamiliar clothes. For many, war work was the first experience they had of wearing trousers. These were a necessity due to the roles women performed in factories.

In Britain in December 1941 the government passed the National Service Act (No 2), which made provision for the conscription of women. Women were required to work in factories or for one of the services. At first only single women and childless widows (aged 20-30) were enlisted into wartime work. But by July 1943 all women aged 31-50 were required to register for war work (many had already voluntarily joined). Women could not serve in active combat, but their varied job roles were hugely important to the war effort.

In Britain and the USA high profile couturiers were asked to design service uniforms. This helped to attract recruits to the various services. In Britain Digby Morton designed the uniforms for the WVS, whilst in America Parisian (yet American-born) couturier Mainbocher designed the uniforms for the Women Accepted for Voluntary Emergency Service (WAVES).

Above: My Great Aunt Thelma was a land girl. Here she is seen wearing a typical land girl uniform including the Land Girl's corduroy breeches.

At the end of the war many women were dismissed from their jobs. Most employers considered that the women were just keeping the jobs ticking over until men returned from active service (some women were allowed to stay on as they were cheaper to employ). However, there were lasting effects. Women had demonstrated that they could do the heavy manual work and within a few decades women in such workforces became a more common sight.

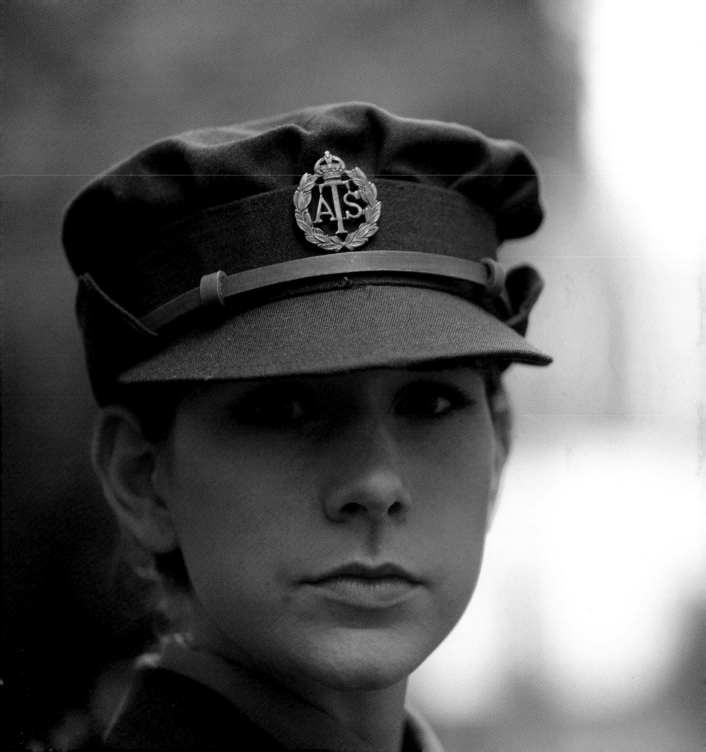

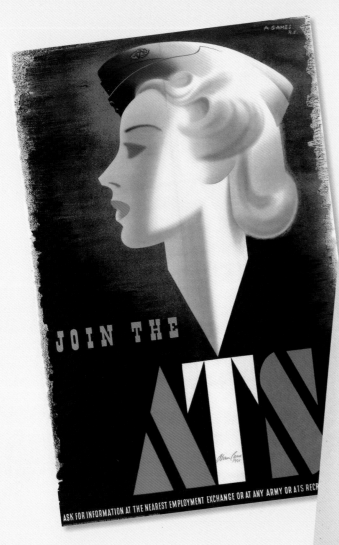

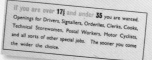

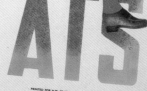

Above and right: Two ATS recruitment posters,
1941 and 1940.

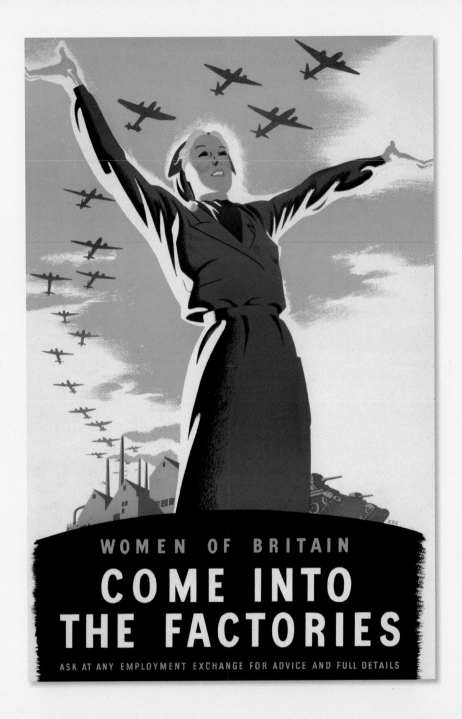

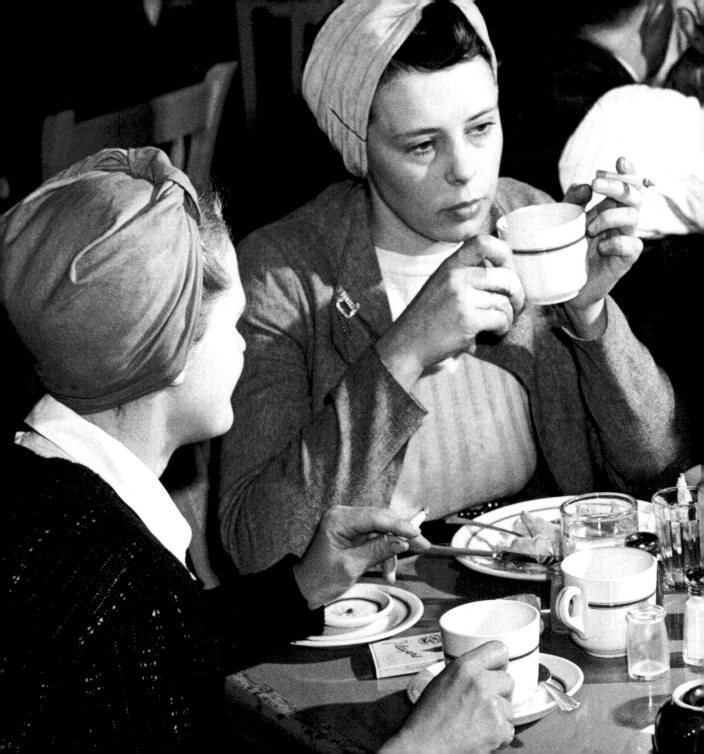

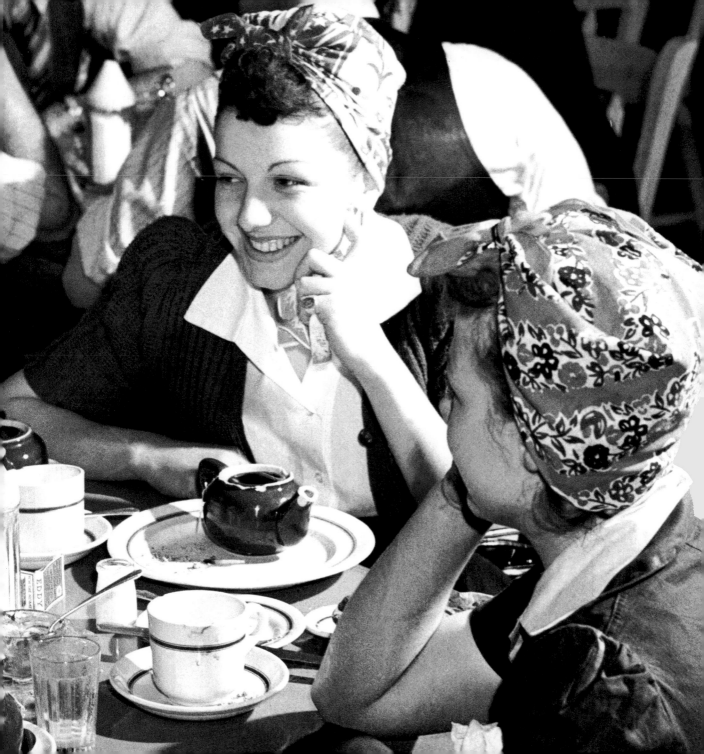

The British Women's Services

- Auxiliary Territorial Service – ATS

Women's branch of the British Army. The first ATS recruits were employed as cooks, telephonists and clerks. By the end of 1941 member's duties were expanded and women worked as drivers, postal workers, radar operators and ammunitions inspectors.

- Women's Auxiliary Air Force – WAAF

Female auxiliary of the Royal Air Force. WAAFs undertook a variety of roles, including compiling weather reports, maintaining aircraft, serving on airfields, operating barrage balloons, parachute packing and working in intelligence.

- Women's Royal Navy Service – WRNS

Female auxiliary of the Royal Navy. WRNS (or Wrens) were females recruited for shore based navy jobs. Wrens played a major part in the planning and organisation of naval operations.

- Women's Voluntary Service – WVS

Initially WVS recruits duties related to the evacuation of children and making medical supplies. Later in the war their duties included salvage and bone collection, running mobile canteen services and providing temporary accommodation for people who had been bombed out of their houses.

- Women's Land Army – WLA

The WLA was created to replace men who had been called up for service and had previously worked in agriculture. Women undertook hard farm work including ploughing, lifting potatoes and lambing.

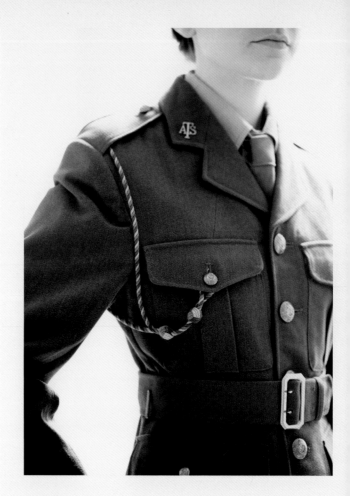

ATS UNIFORM

- Khaki fitted jacked with brass buttons (later changed to Bakelite)
- Paneled khaki skirt with a concealed front pocket
- Khaki shirt
- Dark khaki tie
- Brown flat lace up shoes
- Soft khaki cap

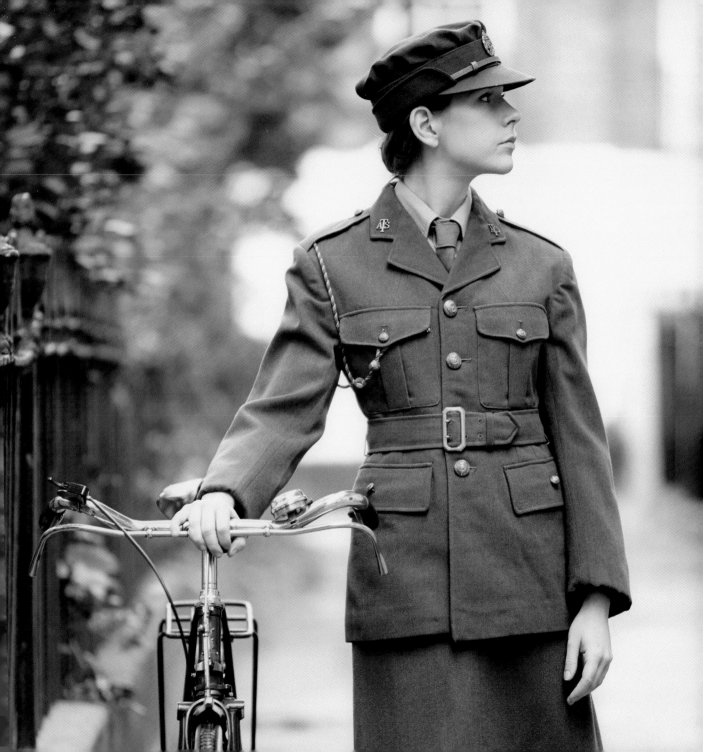

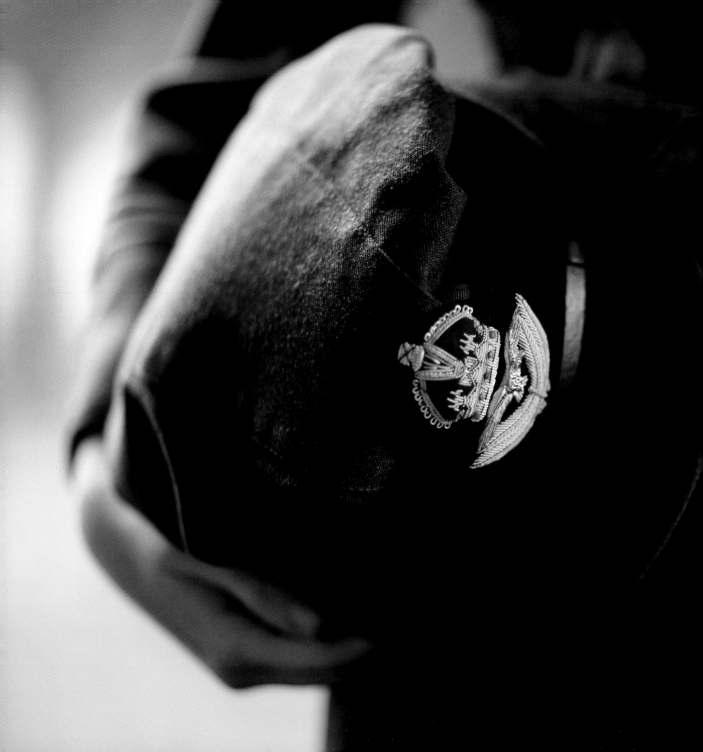

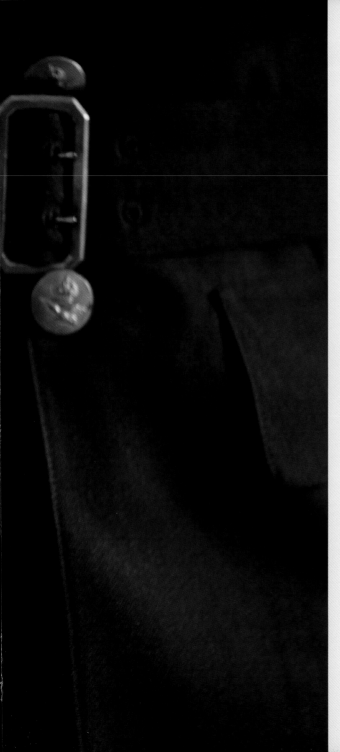

Original uniforms today are highly collectible pieces. If you want to recreate the look there are a number of companies who create accurate reproductions of wartime uniforms (see the reproductions list at the back of the book).

Left: Original WAAF uniform and insignia.

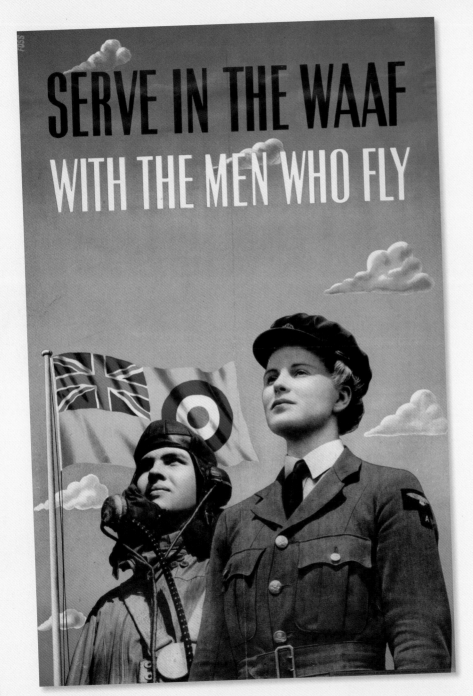

Left: WAAF recruitment poster, 1941.

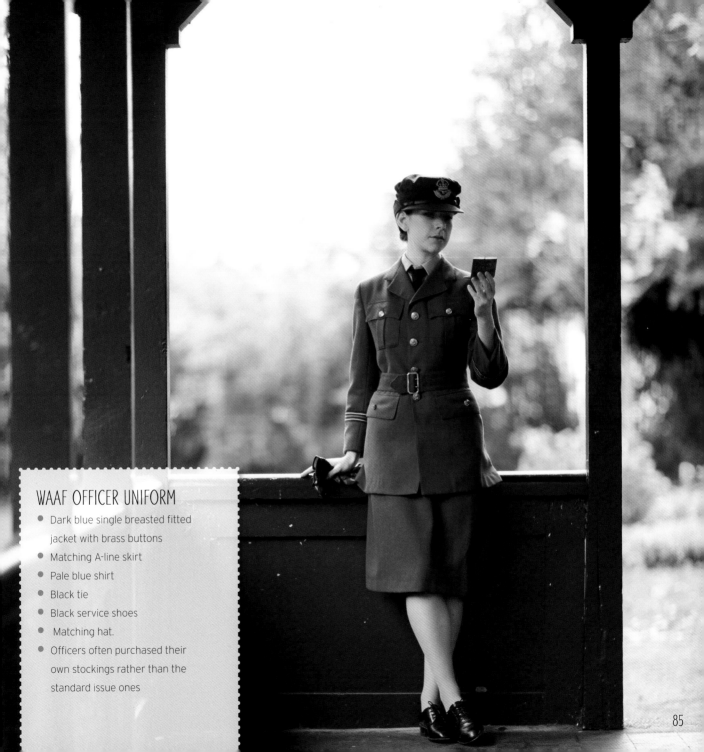

WAAF OFFICER UNIFORM

- Dark blue single breasted fitted jacket with brass buttons
- Matching A-line skirt
- Pale blue shirt
- Black tie
- Black service shoes
- Matching hat.
- Officers often purchased their own stockings rather than the standard issue ones

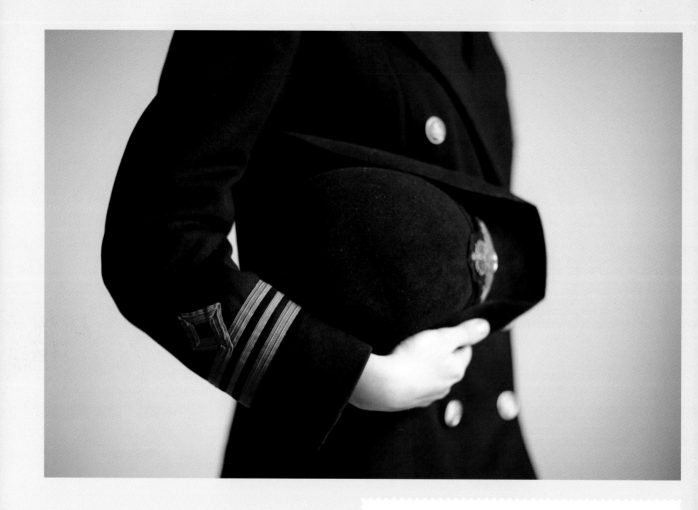

WRNS OFFICER UNIFORM

- Double breasted navy tunic jacket
- Matching A-line skirt
- White shirt
- Navy blue tie
- Black lace-up shoes
- Black lisle stockings (or rayon when they could be obtained)

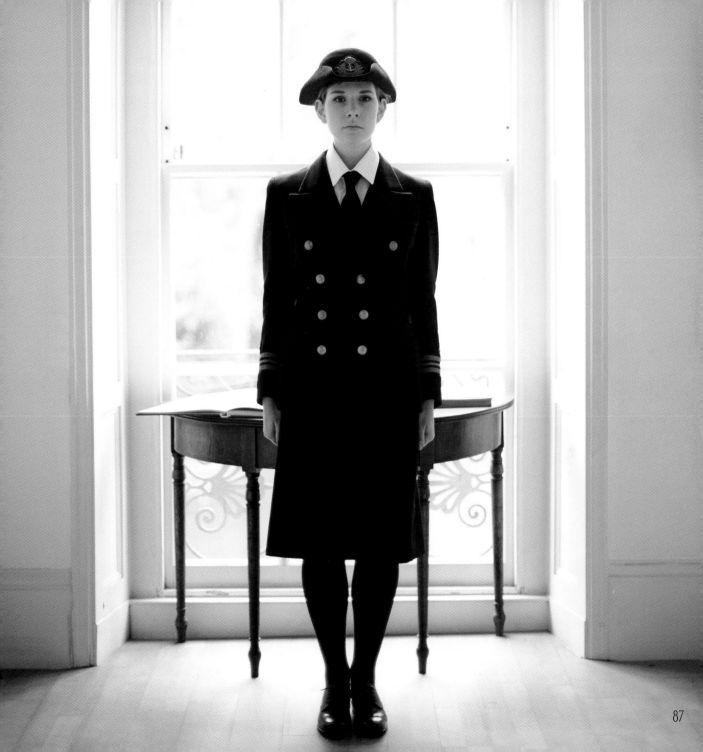

DEVELOPING AMERICAN STYLE

L-85

In 1942 the American War production board introduced a series of rules for the garment industry – 'Limitation orders'. These were directed at restricting manufacturers rather than the general public. It was hoped that the Limitation orders would mean that rationing was not necessary. These orders were the American equivalent of British austerity rulings.

Women's clothing was covered by the order L-85. This altered the silhouette of clothing produced in America, largely affecting the length and sweep of garments. The rulings also dictated things such as depth of hems (no more than 2 inches) and the number of pockets a garment could have (no more than one per blouse/shirt). They were not quite so restrictive as the austerity measures in Britain though. The only people who really suffered with L-85 restrictions were those who were either overweight or very tall.

L-85 restrictions ended in 1946, although the full effects were not felt for consumers until 1947.

American designers really found their feet during the war and developed a style that was identifiably 'American'. Even before the war in America, in particular in New York and California, a unique and successful fashion industry was developing. Where Paris was the centre of couture, New York was fast becoming the centre of Ready-to-Wear (before the 1930s few women had purchased ready made clothing). With the onset of war though, American designers could no longer copy and adapt Parisian designs to suit American tastes, they had to create a look of their own. Two things stand out to me about American wartime fashion– the influence of Hollywood and the development of the casual sportswear industry.

California was the heart of the casual sportswear industry, although sportswear of that time is perhaps not quite what we would consider it today. The casual look consisted of sporty checks for daywear and eveningwear, mix-and-match separates, halternecks, culottes and outfits finished off with flat pumps. Importantly these were garments that were easy to wear.

Right: Holly wears a classic early 1940s burnt orange crêpe day dress. The dress, by American brand Martha Gale, features a faux bolero and feather embroidery to the bust.

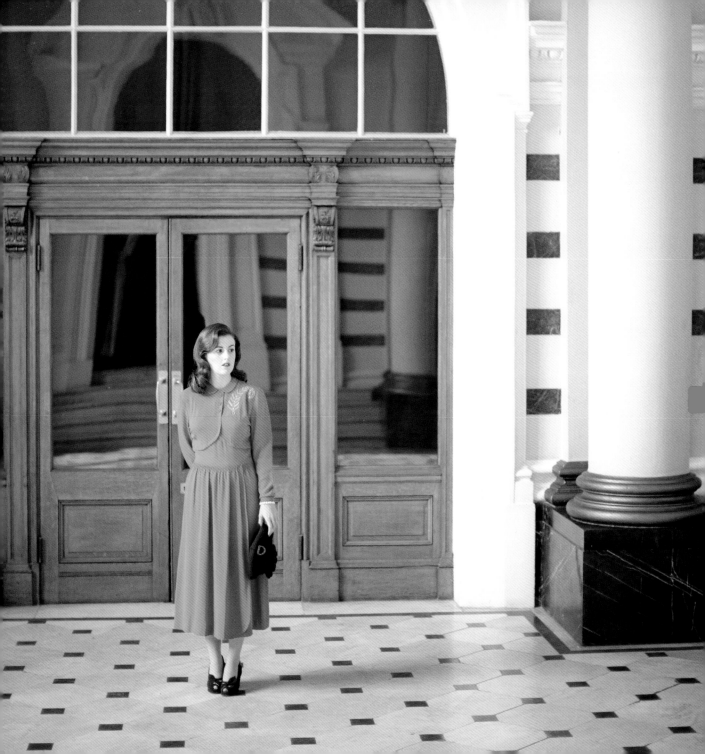

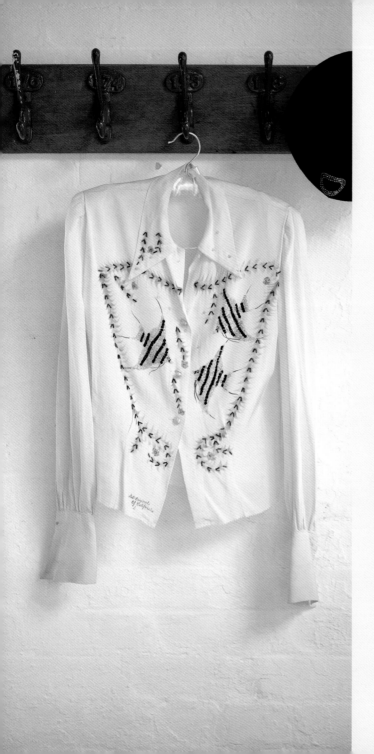

There was also a growing trend towards resort wear. Many American designers, whether they were based in typical resort areas or not, incorporated elements of resort style into their designs – adopting Mexican prints, or the sarong and wrap skirts popular in Hawaii for example.

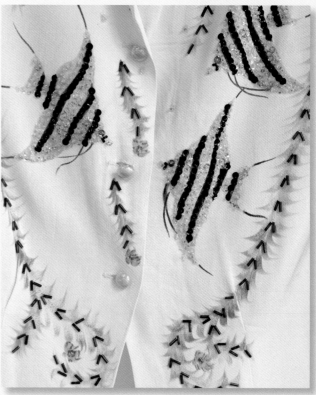

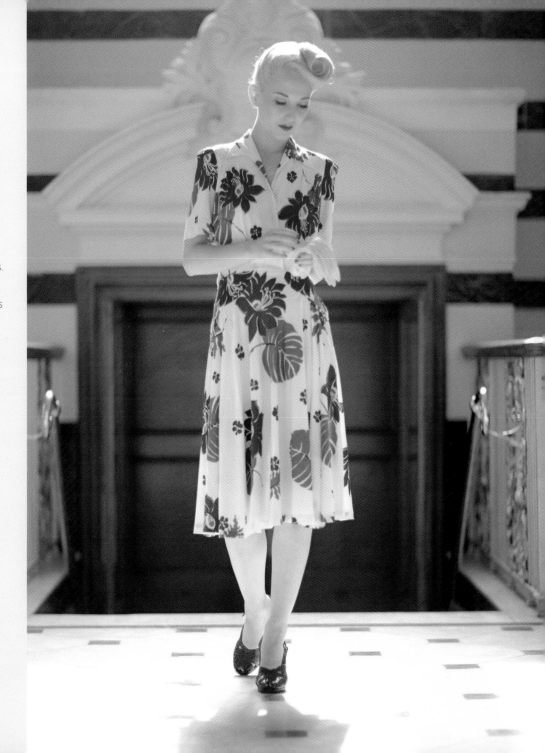

Right: Rosy wears an early 1940s rayon jersey dress printed with Hawaiian motifs.

Opposite: Hand painted blouses were produced in resort areas as souvenir pieces. This sequin embroidered example is signed 'Art Originals of California'.

Hollywood on the other hand represented the glamorous side of the American fashion industry. During the 1930s Hollywood costume designers had already begun to assert their influence upon mainstream designers and this only continued in the 1940s. Designers such as Gilbert Adrian created garments for Hollywood and the American general public. When I think of formal 1940s style it is Adrian's designs (or those inspired by Adrian) that typify the look. Adrian's signature look created a somewhat triangular silhouette: heavily padded shoulders, slimline jackets/dresses placing emphasis across the shoulder, and narrow skirts. His long draped and beaded evening gowns were hugely fashionable, mirroring the style he created on screen.

For me the joy of American wartime clothing is in the clever detailing that remained in them. Long skirts, sweeping dresses with figure-flattering tops, ingenious beadwork and peplums were popular throughout the war and for all levels of the market.

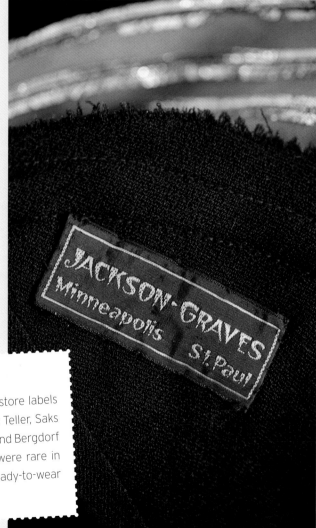

TOP TIP
Keep a lookout for American department store labels from the 1940s. Good ones include Bonwit Teller, Saks Fifth Avenue, Lord & Taylor, Marshall Field and Bergdorf Goodman. Labels crediting the designer were rare in America and most of the successful ready-to-wear designers worked for department stores.

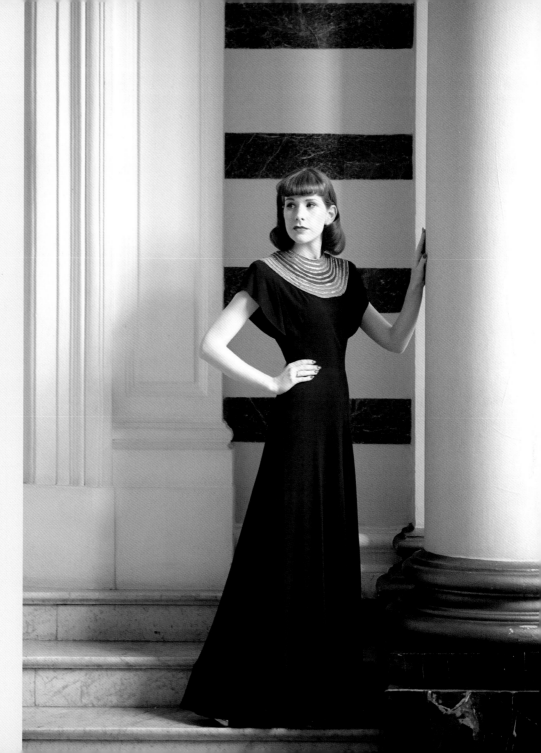

Right: Whilst originals by Adrian are hard to come by, similar American designs can be widely found. This 1940s dress is a personal favourite, made from black crepe it was retailed by Jackson-Graves, a high-end store in Minneapolis. This dress is typical of American evening wear during the 1940s. The dress with its Egyptianesque collar detail features large padded shoulders and a tight nipped-in waist to create a boxy, almost triangular silhouette. Whereas black was rarely seen in British fashion during the war, far more black garments were produced in America where the shortage of dyes was not such a concern.

NEW YORK CREATION

In 1940 a number of fashion professionals in New York came together to try and address how New York could develop its status as a fashion centre to rival Paris. The International Ladies Garment Workers Union and the newly formed New York Dress Institute worked to formulate a plan. They wanted to find a way to promote products made in New York and to increase sales, and so the New York Creation label was born.

As New York was the centre of the American dress trade it was estimated that in 1941 90% of all garments produced would carry the label. The labels were to feature in every garment produced in New York, no matter their cost. This meant that New York Creation labels were found both in simple cotton frocks and elaborate evening gowns too.

There were a number of key attributes that magazines repeated about New York Creation garments; their fit, value, fashion content and craftsmanship.

In 1941 American *Vogue* proclaimed that 'every dress made in New York...every dress no matter what its price...will bear this label. And it is our belief that this labeling, this acceptance of responsibility for the finished product, can not help but stimulate the pride of both manufacturers and workers'.

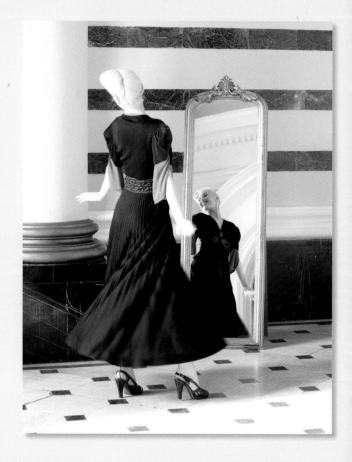

'The latest dresses from New York — where the New begins.'

New York Creation advertising slogan, 1942

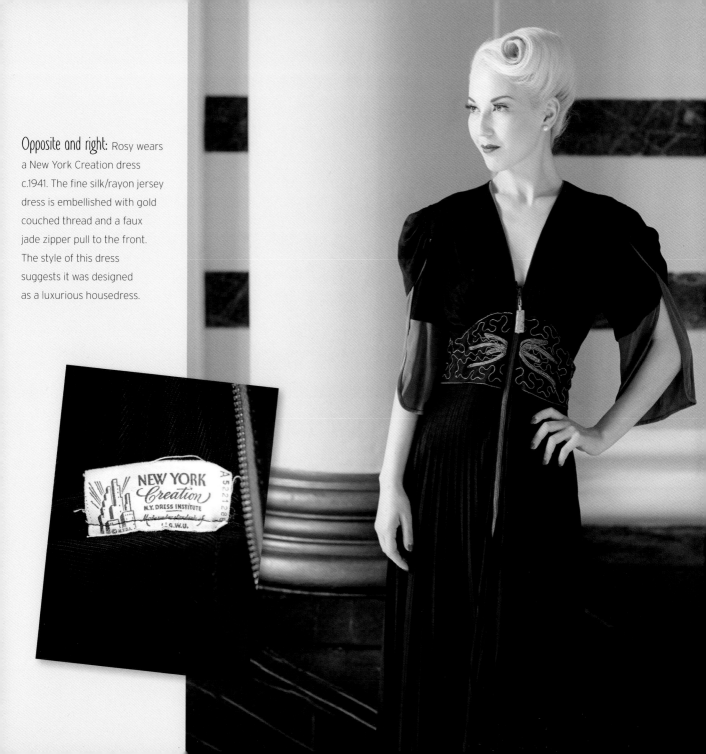

Opposite and right: Rosy wears a New York Creation dress c.1941. The fine silk/rayon jersey dress is embellished with gold couched thread and a faux jade zipper pull to the front. The style of this dress suggests it was designed as a luxurious housedress.

GERMAN STYLE DURING THE WAR

German fashion during the war is often subject to contradicting opinions – whilst a particular image of women was portrayed in German propaganda, all blonde hair and traditional costume, many women did not follow this look, and fashion did still exist in Germany albeit to a limited extent.

Propaganda chief Joseph Goebbels pushed a certain look for German women during the war. Women were expected to be youthful, healthy and natural with scrubbed faces and natural blonde hair. They were meant to wear either the German Dirndl or the Trachtenkleidung (Munich folk costume). This costume generally consisted of a dress or a tight bodice and long full skirt, with white puffy blouse worn underneath, accessorised with an apron embroidered with traditional German motifs.

The dress followed the role desired of German women: the traditional homemaker. Yet, many did not want to submit to this role. Instead they continued wearing clothes with a British, American or French feel to them, and hungrily consumed fashion magazines when they could get their hands on them.

Despite the image Nazi officials wished to portray, wives of the Nazi elite were well known for wearing designer clothing, especially French, and heavy cosmetics.

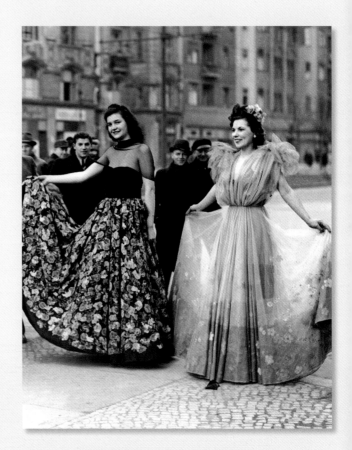

Above: Even after the war German women were facing extreme shortages. This image from 1946 shows two Berliners modelling dresses made from curtain fabric.

Right: Rosy wears an early 1940s German cotton dress printed with traditional motifs.

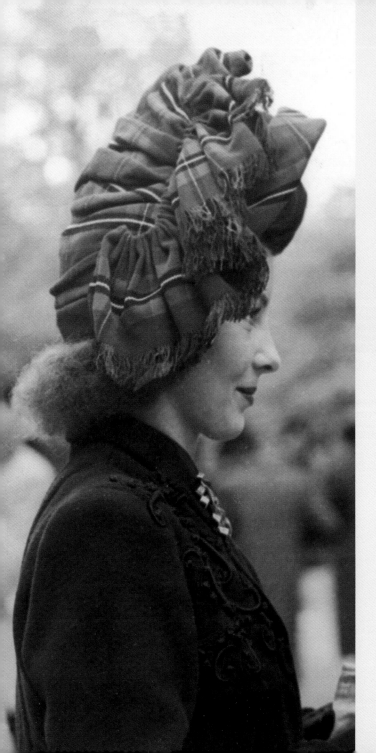

PARISIAN FASHION DURING THE WAR

In June 1940 German forces occupied Paris. It was essential for the city's economic survival that the couture industry was allowed to continue despite the adversity of war and occupation. Fantasy and extravagance continued to dominate French couture despite shortages. Parisian couturiers coped with fabric shortages by making a far smaller number of garments rather than limiting either the workmanship or the amount of fabric that went into each individual garment. Evening dresses looked as if they had been designed for romantic films, with cinched waists and long full skirts.

To ensure that women were still able to purchase couture garments Lucien Lelong (president of the Chambre Syndicale who controlled French couture) negotiated with German authorities. The result was the 'couture card' (plus additional luxury tax). People with a couture card received only half the number of coupons than those who relied upon rationed

Left and right: Parisian women were well known for their elaborate scarf hats. These were created using two or more scarves, lots of false hair and lots of padding.

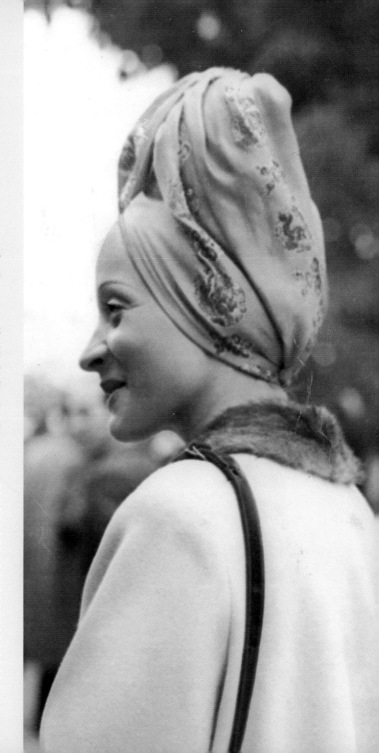

clothes received. They also did not receive coupons with the letter A or B, which French consumers could use to exchange two older garments for one newer one.

Life in occupied Paris for the average woman though was tough, and like her Allied sisters she had to make do with what she could find. Parisian women showed off the Parisienne sense of chic no matter the adversity, making the most of the French rationing system by exchanging old yet wearable garments for new, and re-using old garments in clever ways whenever they could.

Key features of Parisian wartime style

- Extravagant and beautiful hats - pièces de la résistance - demonstrating the imaginativeness and inventiveness of Parisennes.
- Garments similar to British and American, but with more exaggerated elements. Think bigger padded shoulders and more detailing (rouching, draping, exaggerated peplums etc.).
- High clompy shoes, preferably with wooden platforms.

ZAZOUS

The Zazous (or swings) were an early 1940s French subculture. Zazous were young adults aged between 17–20. The subculture was fuelled by swing jazz and bebop music. The men and women involved were well known for their bright, garish and exaggerated clothing.

For women the look tended to consist of a long jacket with heavily padded shoulders and a nipped in waist, pleated skirt and either very flat or very high shoes, often with wooden platforms. The look was accessorised with round, dark sunglasses.

Zazous were well known for their excessive make-up including bright red lipstick. They often dyed their hair blonde and wore it in a style that was raised high above the forehead and fell like a mane down the back. Zazous publicly flouted rationing regulations in France, and the Nazis considered them both decadent and rebellious.

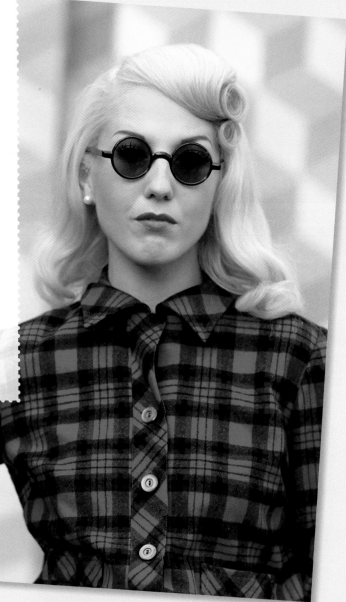

PARIS RE-ASSERTS ITS DOMINANCE

Paris was liberated in August 1944 and the city immediately made plans to recover its status as a fashion capital, although initially couturiers attempts were decidedly rocky. The first collections did not appeal to overseas markets – they were too extravagant and couturiers had to cut back on the material used to meet legal requirements for export. Furthermore, designers were producing a hodgepodge of styles and were not cohesive in the slightest.

The turnaround for Parisian fashion came in 1945 with Théâtre de la Mode. The exhibition borrowed from the 18th century French tradition of dressing dolls in the latest fashions as a promotional tool. The mini mannequins were kitted out to exacting standards in clothing, millinery and accessories. Some seamstresses even crafted miniature undergarments to cover the mannequins modesty. The exhibition opened in Paris in March 1945 and was shown in its entirety in London in the autumn of 1945. Parts of the exhibition travelled to Barcelona, Copenhagen, Stockholm, Vienna and Leeds. In the spring of 1946 the mannequins travelled to New York wearing updated designs reflecting the trends in Parisian fashion to come. The show reminded buyers and consumers alike of the importance of Parisian fashion and was a brilliant PR exercise. It was the perfect taster for the new fashions that would set the fashion world alight in 1947.

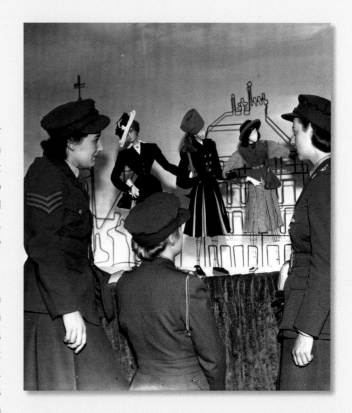

Above: Three ATS girls admiring the Théâtre de la Mode display in London, 1945.

Post-war Fashion

'It's quite a revelation, dear Christian.
Your dresses have such a new look.'

Carmel Snow on Dior's first collection, 1947

In September 1945, World War II officially ended, but this did not bring an immediate change to fashionable dress styles. For many, 1946 was regarded as a war year as far as fashion went – styles remained relatively similar to those during the war and many women were still facing extreme shortages whilst countries recovered financially.

It was not until 1947 that real changes began to occur. Established fashion houses were beginning to get back on their feet and women everywhere were craving something different and exciting – they were craving a *new look*.

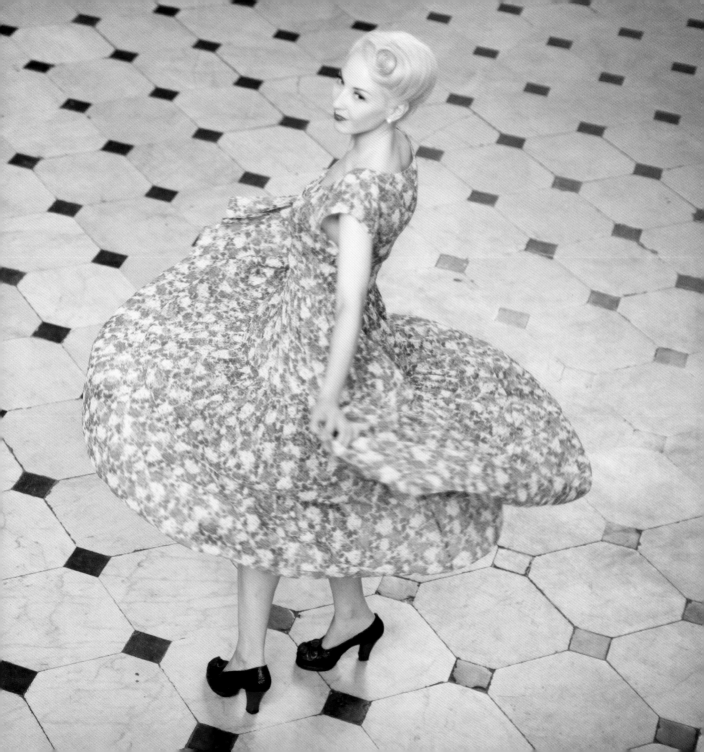

DIOR AND THE NEW LOOK

A few minutes after 10.30am on the 12 February 1947 a new star of Parisian fashion emerged triumphant: Christian Dior. This date saw the unveiling of Dior's first collection, with which he almost singlehandedly turned the fashion world's gaze back to Paris.

However, whilst Dior was shining bright in 1947 he was by no means a new kid on the fashion block, having previously worked for Parisian couturiers Robert Piguet and Lucien Lelong. The turning point for Dior came in 1945, when he was approached by textile magnate Marcel Boussac who enquired if he would like to become the designer for couturier Gaston. Dior did not want to take over an established atelier, his desire was for a small and luxurious fashion house, one that paid homage to the traditions of French superior craftsmanship – combining luxury textiles with complicated cutting techniques and detailed embroidery work. Boussac saw the potential in Dior and agreed to back a new venture – and so the house of Dior was born.

Dior's first collection was named The Corolla, after the inner circle of petals in a flower. Dior was a keen gardener and later went on to suggest that he wanted to create a series of 'women-flowers'. The collection received its nickname 'the New Look' from *Harper's Bazaar* editor Carmel Snow. In fact it might have been more appropriate to call it the old look. Dior's historical references in the collection were plentiful. Whilst Dior suggested that he was heavily inspired by the belle époque, the silhouette of the New Look was also redolent of the mid-19th century crinolines. There were even references to an eveningwear look that some Parisian couturiers had shown in their 1939 collections. By looking to the past for inspiration Dior was seeking to forget the war and return to a time when, in Paris at least, life was calmer, simpler and happier.

This first collection was about making women look like women again – it was swelling, opulent, curving, full and rounded. After years of being trussed up in suits along masculine lines, this style was a chance to revel in the female form. Dior's designs aimed to make women look voluptuous even though many were as thin as rakes owing to wartime food shortages.

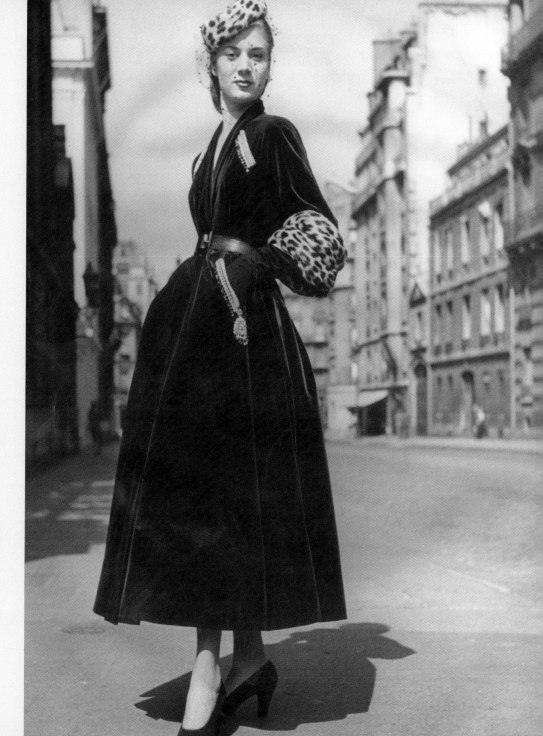

Right: 'Prince Igor', a Christian Dior design as featured in *Picture Post*, September 1947. The outfit consists of a full-skirted green velvet coat with tight belt, gold and silver embroidery over slant pockets and deep leopard skin cuffs. The model wears a matching leopard pillbox hat. This demonstrates the classic Dior silhouette with its nipped in waist and long, full skirt.

The standout piece in Dior's first collection was his infamous Bar Suit. The suit had rounded padded hips, gently padded shoulders, a skirt stiffened with cambric and a tiny nipped in waist. Its finely pleated wool skirt alone contained over 15 yards of material and fell to just 12in above the ground. Many viewed Dior's use of material as excessive, yet not all garments in the first collection included acres of fabric - to please buyers there were narrow skirts and simple suits too.

The New Look celebrated the frivolity of couture. Garments featured complex couture techniques and were labour intensive to create. It was a dreamlike world that Dior had created, but one that many women desired a slice of. Dior's look though was one only afforded by the super rich. The Dior woman epitomised luxury, she had no need to work and was always impeccably groomed. The cost of a Dior gown was inhibitive, even for wealthy women. In 1949 a Dior evening dress cost as much as a new car.

Dior helped to revitalise the Paris fashion industry. Whilst British and American designers were creating their own looks their eyes turned back towards Paris to see the new mode developing. The New Look was lapped up by the international press, but it was not universally popular and it was an adapted version of the style that gained widespread popularity.

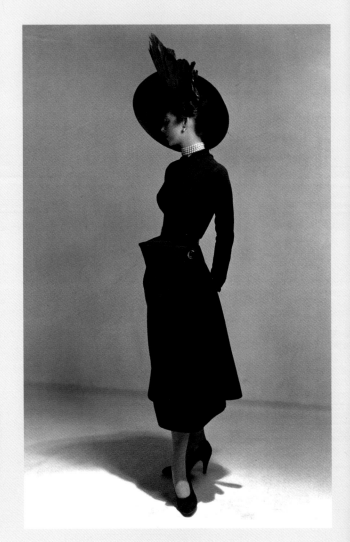

Above: Dress by Christian Dior, 1948.

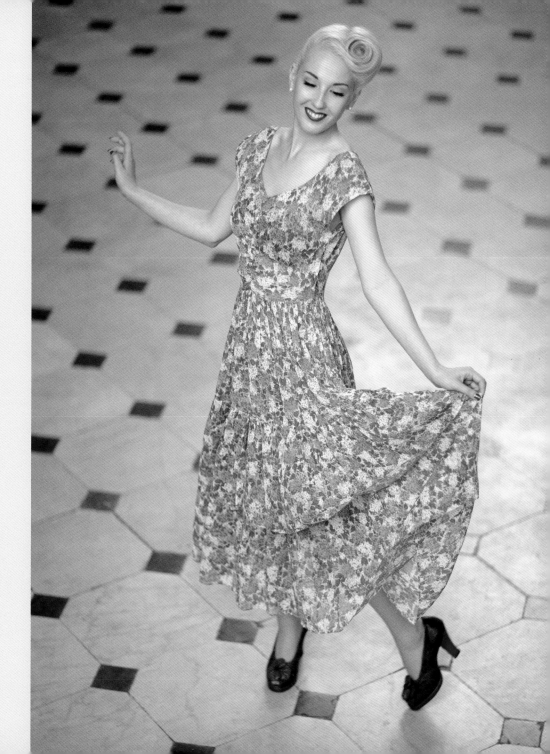

Right: Rosy wears a classic late 40s American voile dress with a very full tiered skirt. This dress demonstrates the more feminine silhouette that was popular after the war.

POST WAR IN BRITAIN AND AMERICA

Whilst Dior helped Paris climb back atop the fashion pyramid, post war there was a thriving fashion industry in existence in both Britain and America. Many of my favourite vintage garments come from the immediate post-war years. Designers still had to deal with restrictions and shortages yet garments feature a more feminine silhouette than those produced during wartime and are both exuberant (and you could say celebratory) in design and colour.

By early 1948 the New Look had taken hold. In April tightly nipped-in waists and longer fuller skirts appeared in London couture collections, whilst ready-to-wear firms such as Cherry were advertising New Look-esque princess coats. They described one of their coats as follows: 'Formal coat elegantly defined in black Barathea. Full, sweeping skirt with the beautiful new parasol here all accentuating the look-how-small waist.'

The Make-do and Mend spirit was not dead in the post-war period. Women who could not afford 'New Look' garments added length to their existing dresses and skirts with trims at the hem, and cinched-in waistlines with belts.

Original photographs from the period demonstrate that, particularly in Britain and America, it was an adapted version of the New Look suited to an active lifestyle that prevailed. Skirts became noticeably fuller and longer, and the masculinity of the overall silhouette was reduced. Yet, many post-war garments in both countries retained the broad shoulder that had been rejected in Paris. Women referred to it as the 'New Look', but it wasn't an exact copy of the design that Dior created.

The combined effects of rationing, utility and austerity had positive results for British manufacturers and consumers alike. Post-war consumers became far more discerning when choosing their clothing – they demanded far better quality ready-made clothing than they had before the war. Furthermore, a new stronger fashion industry was emerging in Britain in the late 40s – one that produced good quality, well designed clothes.

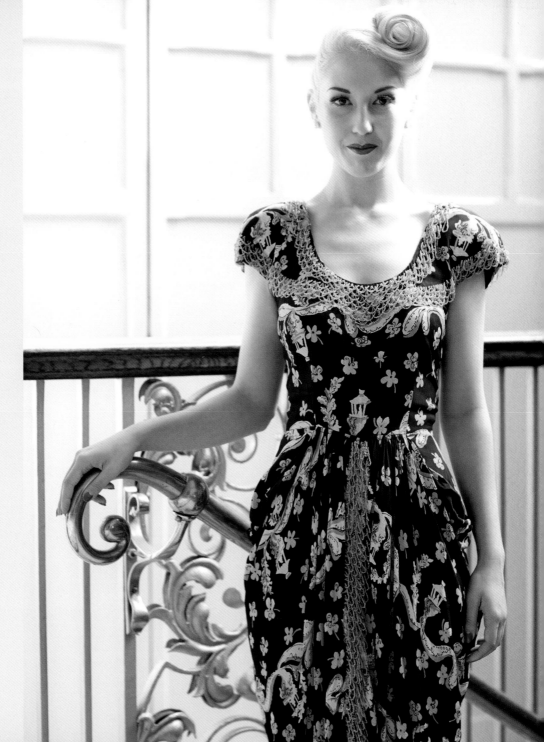

Right: If I had to pick a colour combination that typifies American 1940s design it would be navy blue and pink, and this dress has to be one of the best examples. The dress features rounded shoulder pads and drapery to the front – typical of late 1940s American garments. The pink patterning is perfectly accented with swags of tiny pink seed beads.

Many firms relocated their head offices after being bombed and a number of new firms were also created. The collaborative efforts of designers during wartime only continued post war and a number of groups of ready-to-wear firms formed. In 1946 ten key London firms grouped together to form the Model House Group. This group aimed to increase the export potential of British products through trade shows and selling trips abroad, and also to improve the general standard of ready-to-wear garments.

Whilst British and American designers had been creating their own indigenous looks during the war, post 1947 many turned back to copying or adapting Parisian garments. This was largely a legal business (although there were a number of court cases for illegal copying of Parisian models by American designers!). Designers or owners of ready-to-wear firms would travel to Paris and pay an entry fee to view the couture collections, this would act as a deposit against the purchase of garments. Often one garment purchased would provide ideas for three or perhaps more garments, back in New York or London. These though would have to be edited from the Parisian designs to ensure that they were suitable for the general public and also provided a profit for manufacturers.

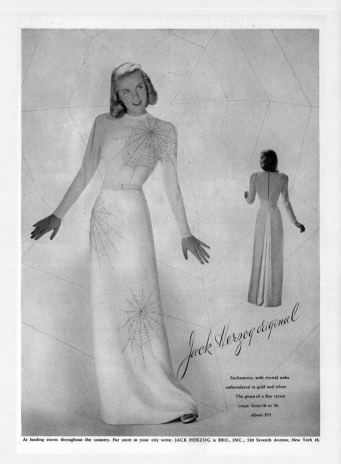

Above: The original advertisement for the dress pictured right.

Right: This rayon crepe dress by New York designer Jack Herzog featured in the August 15 issue of American *Vogue* and it was described as follows: 'enchantress with crystal webs embroidered in gold and silver. Sizes 10-22. About $55.

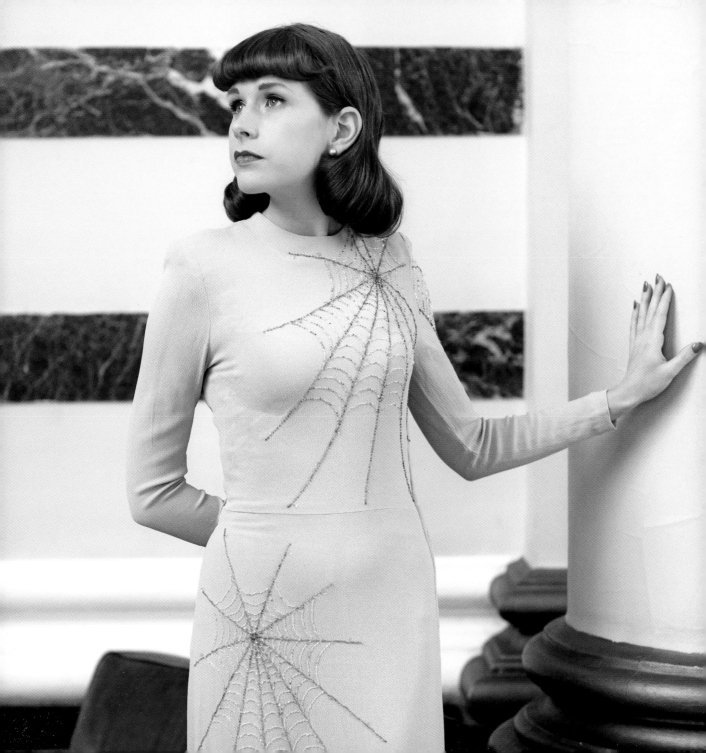

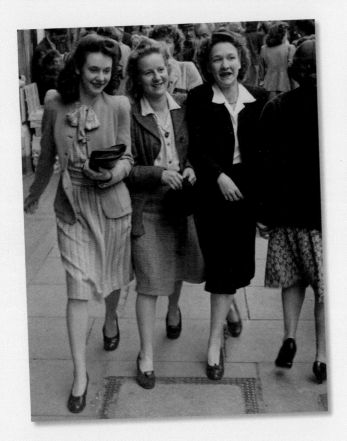

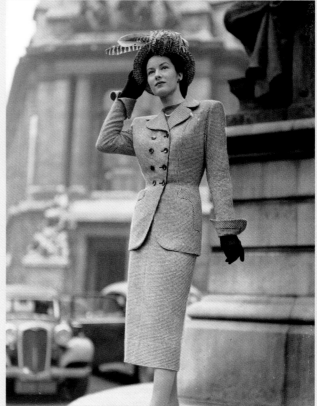

Above left: My Nanna and two friends walking down The Strand in London, July 1946.

Above right: A suit by British ready-to-wear manufacturer Simon Massey, 1947.

Opposite: My Nanna and two friends in St. James' Park in London, August 1947.

LATE 1940S DAYTIME LOOKS

- Calf length skirts
- Exuberant prints
- Nipped-in waists
- Gently padded shoulders
- Dresses in cotton or silk
- Slingback shoes with peep toes
- Belted wool coats with pleated skirts
- Small neat hats and matching gloves.

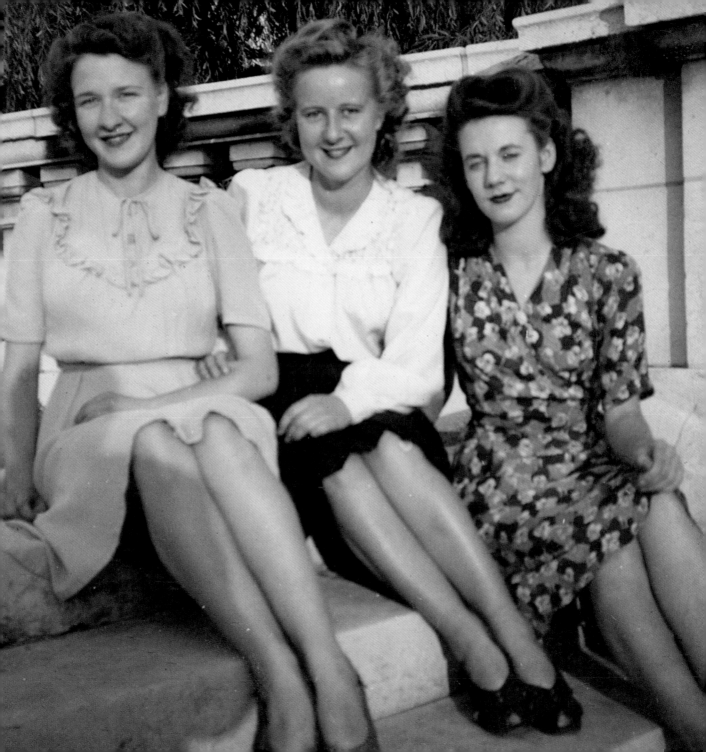

BRAND SPOTLIGHT
LILLI ANN

When hunting for vintage suits look out for this brand – Lilli Ann epitomise the height of American style. The company was founded in 1933 in San Francisco by Adolph Schuman and soon became recognised for their expertly crafted, often elaborately designed, smart suits. Good Lilli Ann suits can command huge sums today, although it should be noted that they were very expensive when new. Whereas a lovely wool crêpe suit from the Sear's catalogue might have cost you $20 in the late 40s, a Lilli Ann would likely have cost around $100.

Right: Rosy wears a Lilli Ann suit in black boucle wool with Canadian lynx fur cuffs. The firm were producing similar suits to this during the 1950s too.

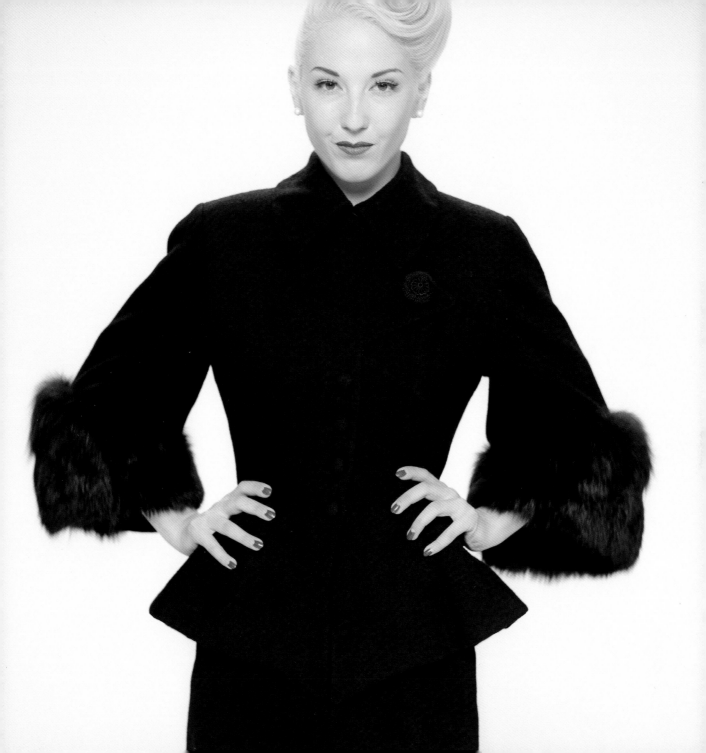

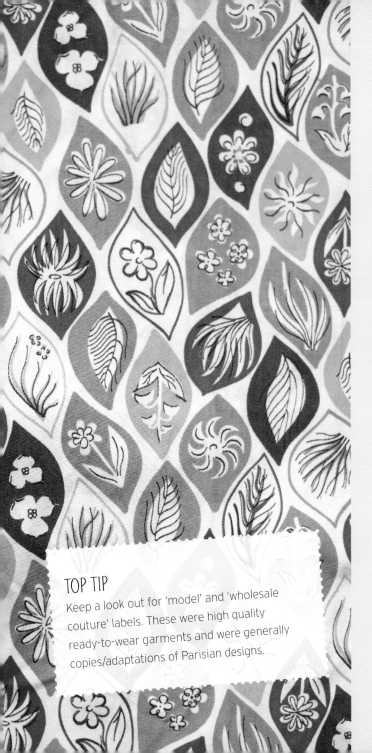

POST-WAR BRITISH LABELS TO LOOK OUT FOR

All of these firms were producing high quality garments straight after the war. It should be noted that many firms were still operating well into the 60s and even 70s.

- Frederick Starke
- Dorville
- Matita
- Koupy
- Susan Small
- Brenner
- Frank Usher
- Doree Leventhaal
- Elizabeth Henry
- Hershelle
- Dereta
- Simon Massey

TOP TIP
Keep a look out for 'model' and 'wholesale couture' labels. These were high quality ready-to-wear garments and were generally copies/adaptations of Parisian designs.

Left and opposite: A selection of exhuberant late 40s fabrics.

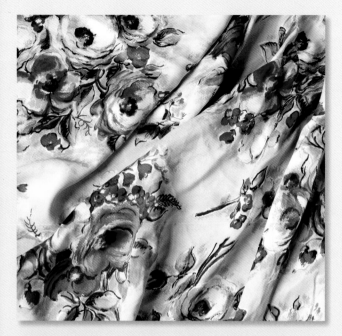
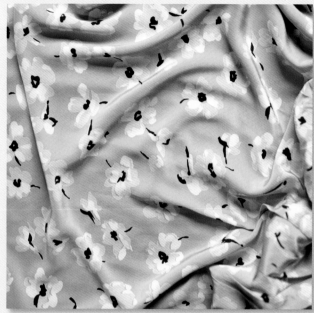
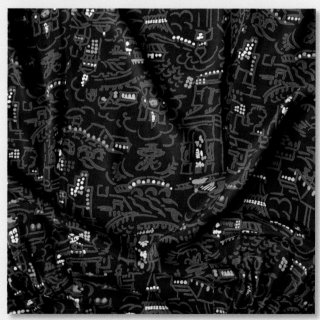
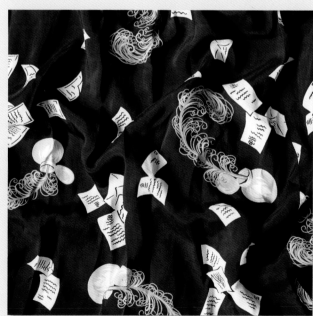

117

BRAND SPOTLIGHT
HORROCKSES

The history of Horrockses stretches back to 1791, when the firm was established in Preston, Lancashire. Horrockses developed a reputation as a textile manufacturer producing high quality cotton to be sold on to garment producers, or used for things such as bed sheets, towels and tablecloths. The fashion branch of the business, Horrockses Fashions was established in 1946 as a vehicle to promote their superior cottons.

Horrockses quickly became associated with bold floral prints, bayadère stripes and intriguing novelty designs. Importantly Horrockses garments were all produced using their own cotton with special finishes that helped garments to last longer. Many women who wore the dresses in the 40s and 50s testify to the fact that they could be cleaned and pressed time and time again without damaging the robust fabric.

Horrockses dresses were mass-produced, but they still aimed for an air of uniqueness within their garments. The prints were almost always exclusive to the brand and all designs were produced in limited runs.

Pieces by Horrockses are highly desirable in the collectors' market, especially when the print designer can be identified. Horrockses regularly advertised in major magazines such as *Vogue* and *Ambassador,* making it easier to date their garments.

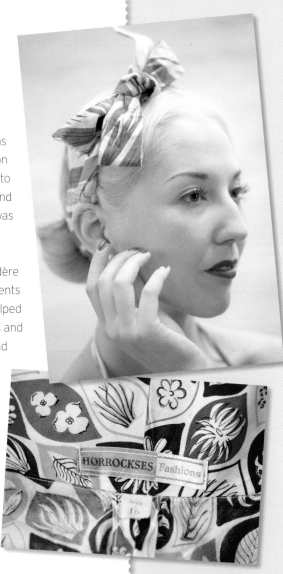

Right and opposite top:
This Horrockses dress with
matching bolero jacket and
headscarf was featured in
Vogue in May 1948. Retailed
exclusively by Harvey Nichols,
the dress cost £5 7s. 8d.
and required 10 coupons.
The print was designed by
Alastair Morton.

Bottom left: Late 1940s
Horrockses garments contain
a printed label. From the early
1950s onwards Horrockses
began producing garments
with a woven label.

It's all in the detail

jewellery, shoes and handbags

'It is wise to buy good accessories, for nothing, cheapens an outfit so much as tawdry trimming.'

The Guardian, 24 April 1940

The 1940s represents a decade of intense creativity as far as accessories went. Women everywhere were creating accessories with whatever they could find, whether this meant creating jewellery from wire and wood or handbags from crochet and felt. Scraps of fabric, however tiny, would be turned into inventive brooches or used as appliqués on bags and belts.

It was not only women at home who got inventive though, designers did too. Shoe designers created vertiginous heels using everything from cork to straw, whilst jewellers were using offcuts of Lucite to create novelty pieces.

Accessories during the decade were used by women to brighten up tired clothes past their best and ensured women looked presentable despite the shortages they faced.

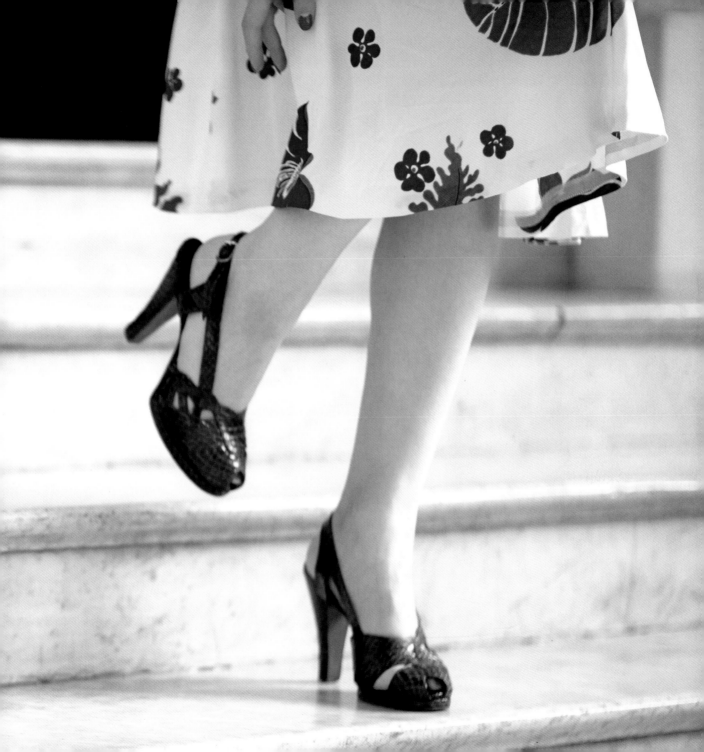

JEWELLERY

During the war, with clothes shortages at their height, jewellery remained exuberant and acted as the perfect tonic to brighten up any dull, tired or shabby outfit.

At the beginning of the war regimental and insignia badges were hugely popular throughout the allied countries. These were often made from metal and sometimes set with marcasite and precious stones. By 1942 in the UK most metal jewellery had ceased to be produced (ID bracelets, cufflinks and wedding rings were still being produced in small numbers). The reasons for this were threefold: the bombings decimated jewellery manufacturing centres such as Birmingham; those jewellery factories that survived were often converted into sites for the manufacture of bullets and radio parts; and finally metal was desperately needed for the war effort.

There was a strong market in Britain for second-hand and antique jewellery because it was so difficult to buy new. Lots of pieces were broken down and re-set to make attractive new pieces. As with clothes, women got inventive and tried making jewellery out of all sorts of weird and wonderful materials (anyone for jewellery made from cutlery?). Wood, wire, oddments of plastic and felt were the most common materials used for homemade pieces in Britain.

I must admit, that in terms of 1940s jewellery, it is the costume pieces produced in America that really set my heart racing. The outbreak of World War II left America isolated from Europe and not only did designers begin creating their own indigenous style in terms of clothes, but in jewellery too. Whereas the French jewellery industry was just about surviving, the American one was thriving. Designers in America had to be inventive though, as they could not import raw materials, such as rhinestones from Czechoslovakia or Austria, on the scale needed.

American costume jewellers substituted sterling silver for base metals and swapped European paste and gemstones for new plastics such as Lucite. The Americans perfected coating sterling silver with a thin layer of gold plate to create vermeil – easily mistaken for real gold. These pieces were often set with clashing combinations of enormous faux gems – aquamarine and ruby red for example.

Right: A late 40s bracelet and ring. The ring features a large Czech glass stone, but the ring was likely produced in America.

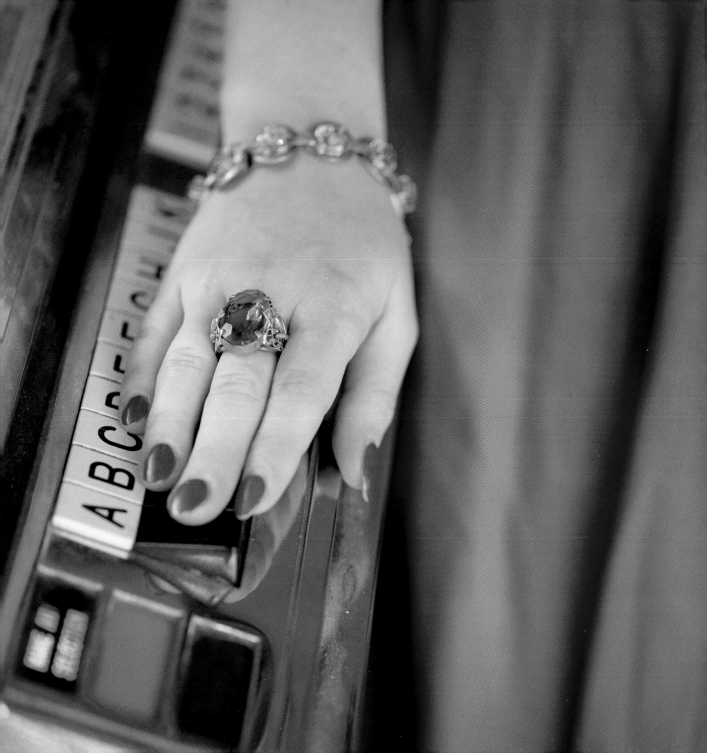

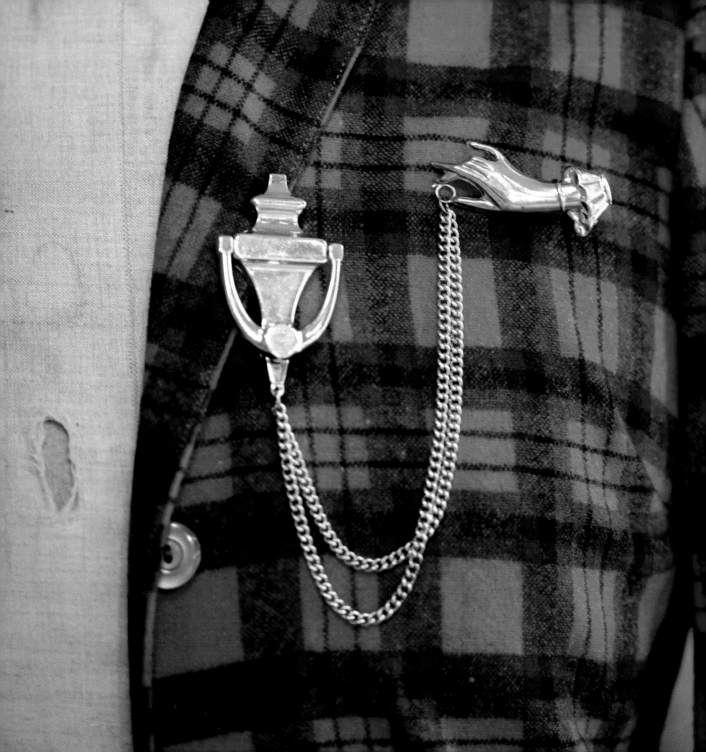

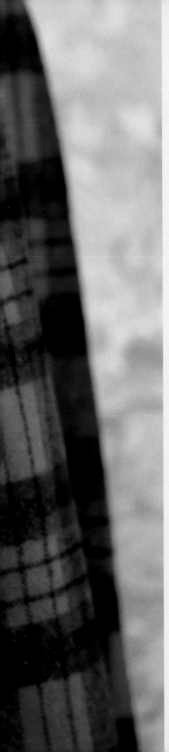

BRAND SPOTLIGHT
CORO

Coro was established in 1901, and during the 1940s was regarded as both an imitator and an innovator in terms of jewellery production. At the height of the company's production in the 30s and 40s Coro employed nearly 3500 staff and had factories in the USA, Canada and Britain. The prolific output meant that Coro produced styles at every quality level and for every budget.

Design director Adolph Katz joined the firm in 1924 and spearheaded the company's rapid expansion. Katz was well known for his whimsical style and was responsible for a number of hugely successful pieces, including his *en tremblant* floral pins (in which a flower is mounted on a spring so that it trembles when the wearer moves), friendship sets and Coro Duettes.

Coro produced a number of different lines. The standard Coro line was of good quality, whilst the Corocraft range (introduced in 1937) targeted the higher end of the market. Other lines produced by Coro include Vendome (introduced in 1944) and Pegasus (introduced post-WWII).

Left: This large doorknocker duo brooch was designed by Adolph Katz c.1945 and doubles as a cardigan clip. This piece comes from the Coro Pegasus range. The hand motif has several historical references calling to mind the Victorian era and surrealism.

BRAND SPOTLIGHT
TRIFARI

Italian immigrant Gustavo Trifari established the brand Trifari in New York c.1910 and it wasn't long before Trifari became one of America's leading costume jewellery manufacturers. The brand received extensive publicity and had a glittering list of exclusive clientele who valued their high quality, well-designed costume pieces. Alfred Phillipe was the company's chief designer between 1930 and 1968 and was well known for his realistic imitations of precious jewellery crafted in materials such as silver, Lucite, rhinestones and faux pearls.

During WWII, Trifari began producing Lucite windshields and turrets for American fighter planes in some of its factories. The rejects and offcuts were discarded until someone (possibly Phillipe) came up with the ingenious idea of cutting the discarded Lucite into cabochons and using them as the 'bellies' for their animal pins. These Lucite bellies can be found in a whole range of animals from seals to roosters, although poodles are especially rare and coveted by collectors.

Opposite: Trifari were widely copied. Coro for example released their own versions of Trifari's jelly bellies. The crown was one of Trifari's signature motifs and their crown brooch was devised in 1941. Trifari crowns are somewhat fanciful and tend to feature jarring combinations of gems in red, green and deep blue. This crown pin is unmarked, but copies the Trifari style.

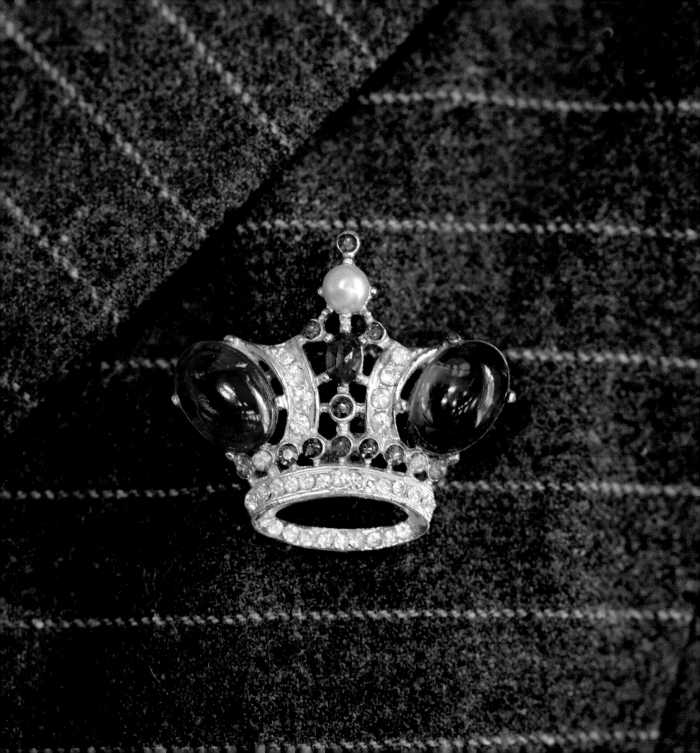

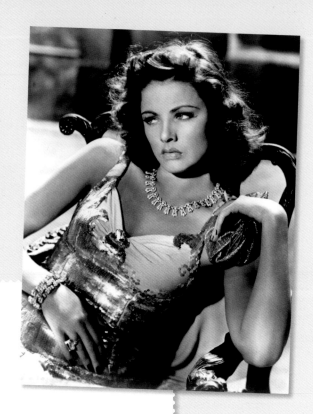

BRAND SPOTLIGHTS
JOSEFF OF HOLLYWOOD

Joseff of Hollywood costume jewellery has to be the epitome of silver screen glamour. Joseff abandoned a successful career in advertising to pursue his passion: costume jewellery. In the 1930s he became a leading supplier of costume jewellery for major film studios and by the 40s he was supplying over 90% of the jewellery in Hollywood films. 1940s films featuring his jewellery included *Down to Earth*, *Ziegfeld Follies* and *The Three Musketeers*. Joseff developed fantastic research skills during his career in advertising and this helped him to create accurate replicas of historical pieces for film. These pieces proved so popular with the film stars that he began producing them for the commercial market. Joseff was well known for creating 'Russian gold' a matte, camera-friendly alternative to gold. His pieces, especially those in Russian gold, are highly sought after by collectors.

Above: Actress Gene Tierney wearing Joseff of Hollywood jewellery in *The Shanghai Gesture*, 1941, directed by Josef Von Sternberg.

Opposite: Patriotic jewellery was worn by women around the world to show their support for the war. This American Eagle was produced in America in the early 1940s.

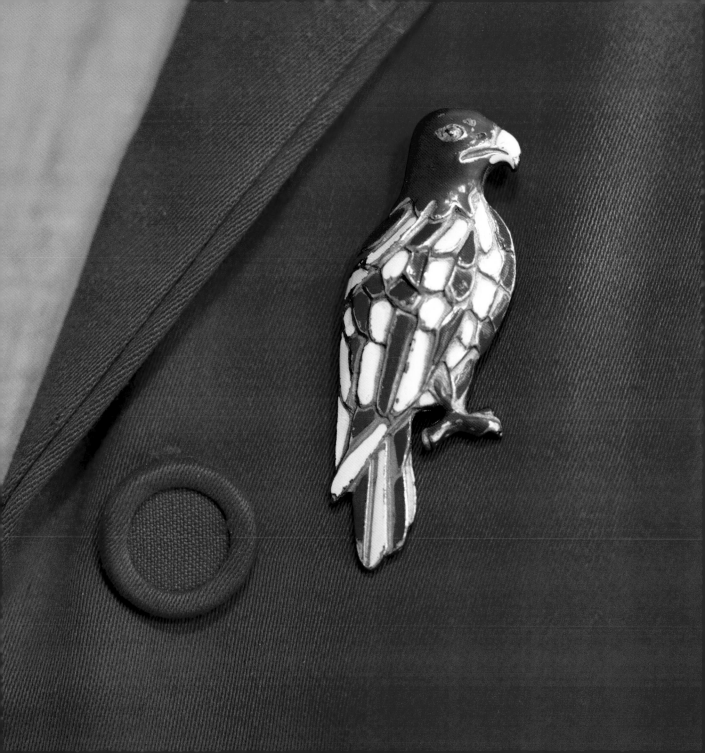

BAKELITE

Bakelite jewellery had been popular during the 1930s, but in the 1940s its popularity soared even further. Designers created fantastical novelty pieces resembling everything from fruit to hearts and even to animals.

Martha Sleeper was one such producer of novelty Bakelite pieces. Sleeper had been a silent film star in the 20s and 30s but in the 1940s made a step in to jewellery design. She created whimsical pieces in not only Bakelite, but also wood and metal. Her designs included everything from Bakelite elephants brooches to back-to-school charm bracelets.

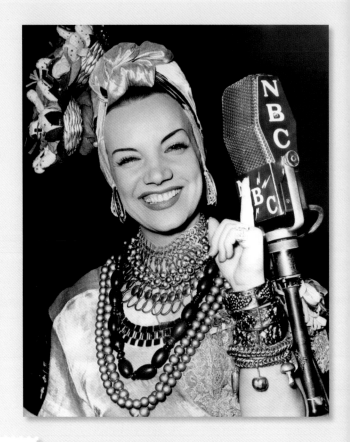

Above: Carmen Miranda was well known for her extravagant jewellery. Here she is seen wearing numerous strings of colourful beads, likely made from Bakelite.

OTHER BRANDS TO LOOK OUT FOR

- Kramer, established in New York in 1943
- Jomaz (Joseph J Mazer & Co), established in New York in 1946
- Miriam Haskell opened her first jewellery shop in 1924. Her company's designs used high quality materials, including Murano beads and Austrian glass crystals
- Weiss, established by Albert Weiss (a former Coro designer) in 1942

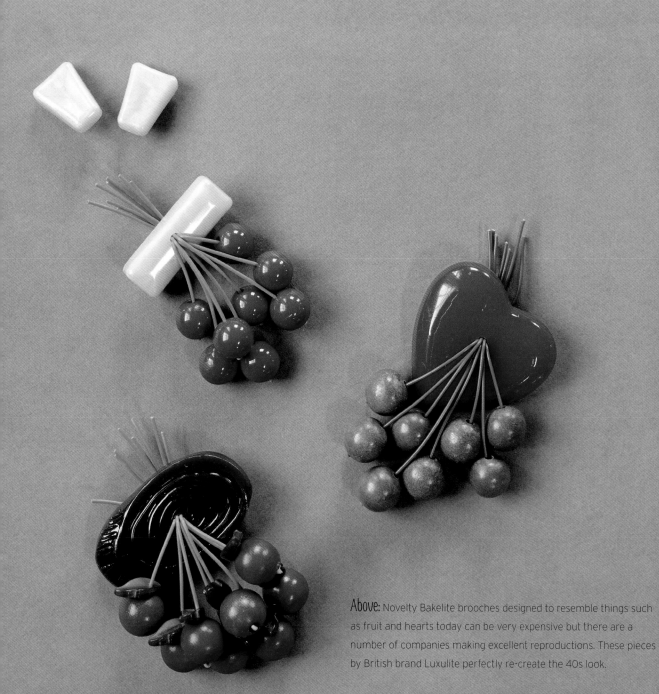

Above: Novelty Bakelite brooches designed to resemble things such as fruit and hearts today can be very expensive but there are a number of companies making excellent reproductions. These pieces by British brand Luxulite perfectly re-create the 40s look.

SHOES

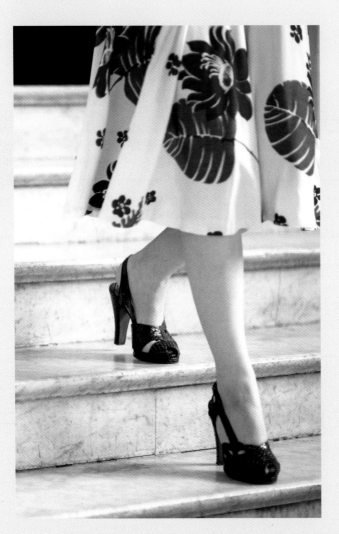

The 1940s was undeniably the decade of the platform. In France during the occupation women's platform shoes reached vertiginous heights with at least 2 inch platforms and 4 inch heels. In both America and Britain platform shoes were popular too, but not as high as the French examples! There were lots of varieties of the platform shoe. Some came with platforms covered in fabric, others with contrasting cork or wood platforms. The bifurcated wedge was an alternative to the platform – effectively a full wedge in which there is only a tiny gap between the platform sole and the heel. Platform shoes were worn until the 1950s in both America and Britain, but their popularity waned in France as they were considered to be symbols of the occupation.

For everyday wear most women chose masculine looking shoes for practical reasons, selecting designs that were hardwearing and built to last. The leather brogue was hugely fashionable with either full front or short side laces, and sometimes with suede accents.

Left: A pair of late 1940s green lizard slingback sandals.

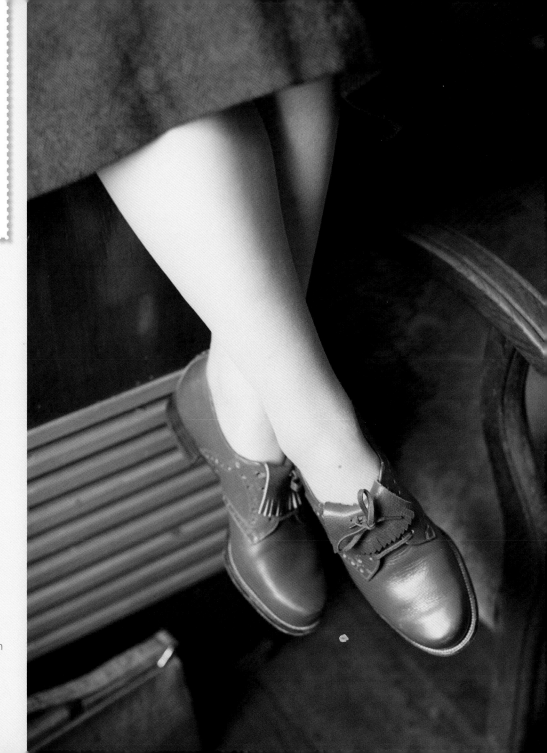

TOP TIP
A modern pair of classic plain brogues in navy or tan leather (as long as they have leather soles) can recreate the look of original 40s brogues effectively.

Right: A pair of chestnut brown leather brogues featuring the CC41 stamp.

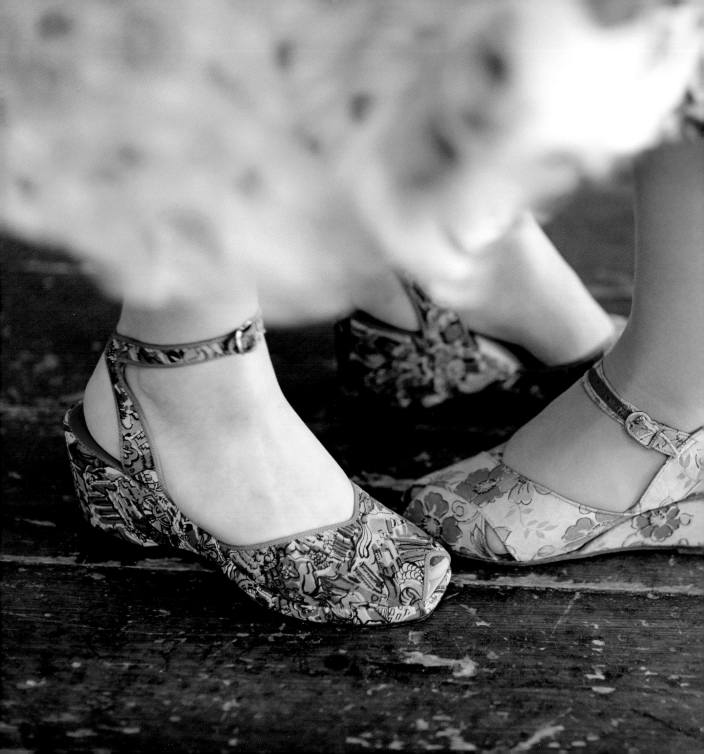

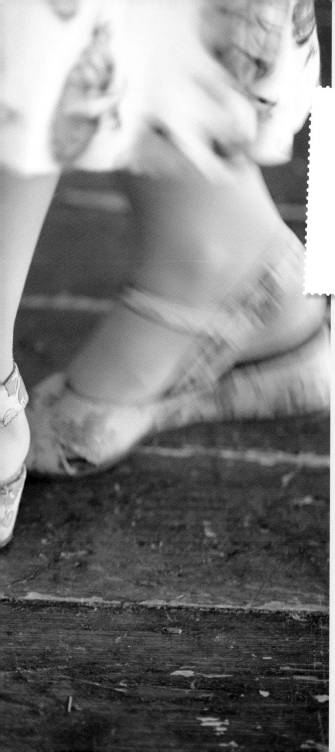

1940S SHOE STYLES AND FEATURES

- Lace-ups
- Spectator shoes
- Platforms and wedges
- Rich vibrant colours
- Wood and cork
- Resort sandals.

Left: Summer sandals from different continents. A pair of early 1940s American rayon sandals and a pair of early 1940s British cotton sandals. Both have wooden heels.

Owing to leather shortages, shoes in the 40s were often made from non-traditional materials. Innovative designers such as Andre Perugia and Salvatore Ferragamo used all sorts of unusual materials for their shoes including woven straw, raffia, plaited cellophane, tree bark, hemp, paper, cork and even fish skin.

Shoes with wooden soles were seen during the war in Europe and America. Examples covered with fabric, rather than plain wooden heels, were most popular. Clogs (sabots in France) were repeatedly promoted during the war, but they never really caught on as a true fashion item.

Post-war, shoe styles changed only slightly from those worn during the war. Gradually more feminine styles were worn in Europe and America. Shoes showed off elegant feet, heels became slightly slimmer and peep toes grew marginally larger placing more of the foot on display.

BRANDS TO LOOK OUT FOR

- Brevitt
- Lilley and Skinner
- Bective
- Bally
- Lotus
- Rayne
- Holmes
- Joyce
- Church's
- Selby
- Gold Cross

DID YOU KNOW?

The only items that were rationed in the USA were leather shoes – every person was allowed three pairs per year, which in fact was roughly the average purchased anyway. Women in America could however purchase leather-soled textile shoes and also cork, straw, wood and rope-heeled shoes.

Right: A pair of mid-1940s platform shoes by British brand Lotus. The shoes are made from high quality thick leather.

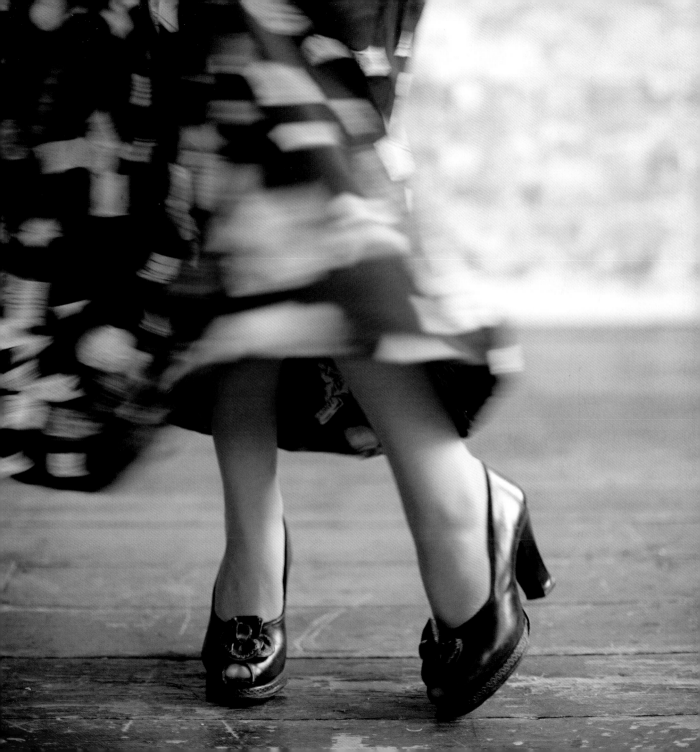

HANDBAGS

During WWII the essential characteristic that all handbags required was practicality. Military influenced satchels with sturdy thick straps and buckled flaps were therefore de rigeur. Many women chose to carry shoulder bags as opposed to hand-held bags due to their practicality.

The interior of handbags changed during the war as mirrors disappeared from inside them. Zips and clasps were rarely made from metal, as it was needed for the war effort.

Around the world women were creating homemade handbags, often from materials such as felt, string and raffia. Raffia was a favoured material as it created both decoration and structure. Homemade envelope clutches, pouches and reticules executed in bright colours could liven up any outfit.

Handbags were often given as low price homemade gifts during the war. British *Vogue*'s 1942 Christmas issue advocated making a chunky suede pouch, 'a bigger and better version of last war's Dorothy bag to hang like a big bow from your wrist.'

After the war ended there was a decided change back towards smaller daintier handbags – ladylike bags reigned again. The shoulder bag was largely relegated and women reverted to the classic handbag.

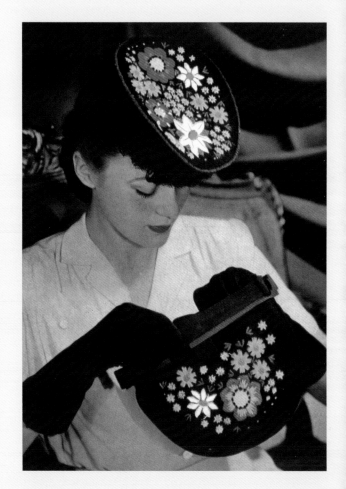

Above: Matching knitted hat and handbag embroidered with a floral design, from a knitting pattern booklet, 1946.

Right: Accessories featuring corde decoration (finely twisted braid) were produced both in American and Britain. This corde handbag is American, whilst the shoes are British.

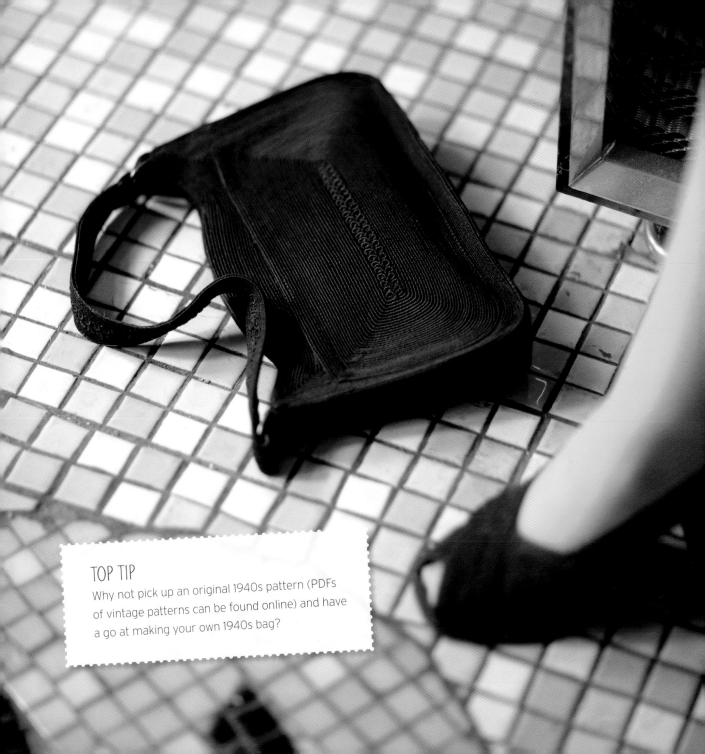

TOP TIP

Why not pick up an original 1940s pattern (PDFs of vintage patterns can be found online) and have a go at making your own 1940s bag?

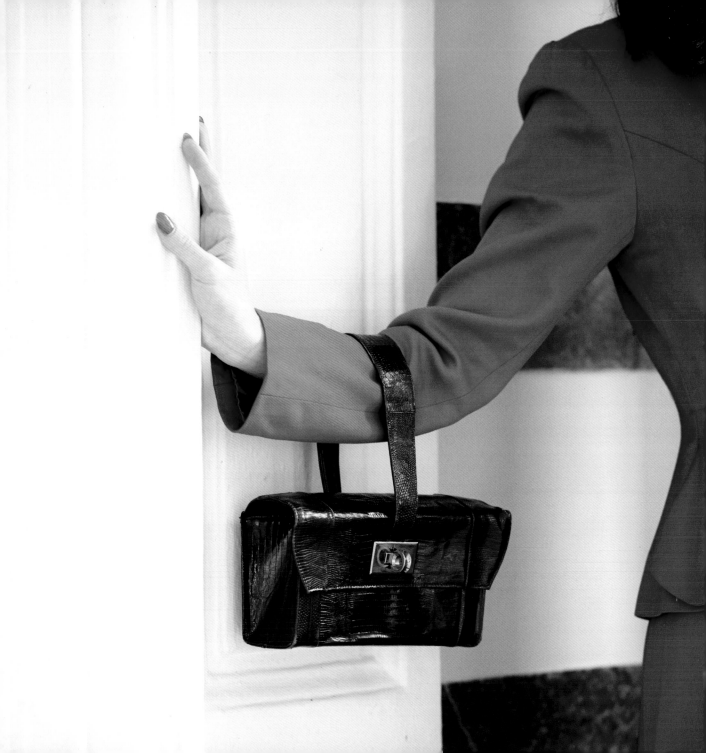

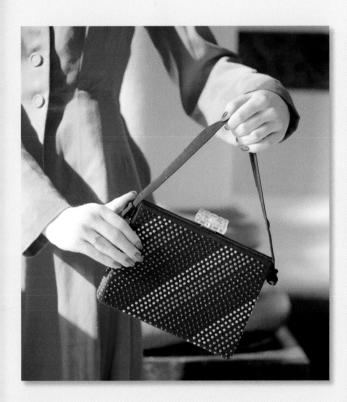

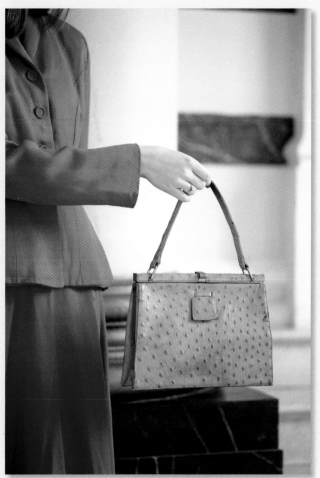

Above: This handbag is typical of the exuberant handbags produced in America, with its raised blob decoration and Lucite clasp. Towards the end of the 1940s handbag manufacturers such as Rialto, Llewelyn and Gilli originals were getting imaginative with their bags and started to craft entire handbags out of Lucite.

Left: Wristlet handbags were popular for evening throughout the 1940s. This early example is made from lizard skin.

Above: Handbags in exotic skins such as ostrich were used for daytime during the 1940s. This example is lined in butter soft leather – a sign of a high quality product.

Lingerie and swimwear

'Jantzen makes the whole world swim.'

Jantzen advertising slogan, 1947

The 1940s was a decade of increasing brevity in both swimwear and lingerie. Both were getting smaller – with brassieres reduced to two triangles of fabric and swimsuits increasingly two-piece as opposed to one.

Lingerie was first and foremost a practical concern. Most lingerie throughout the decade needed to create shape under a garment and in the cold winters of wartime keep a woman warm. Vests were therefore a necessary for many women. Underwear was always in fleshy neutral tones, beiges, pinks and white, and often finished off with delicate lace or sprigs of floral embroidery. No bright colours were allowed!

Swimwear however was exuberant throughout the decade and swimsuits and two-pieces were often seen in bold clashing primary colours and riotous prints.

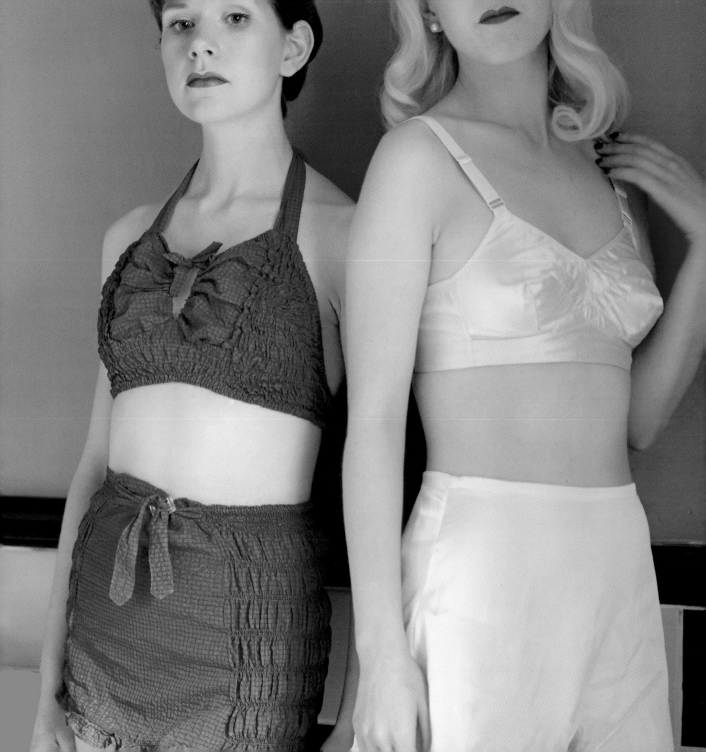

LINGERIE AND LOUNGEWEAR

Women's underwear during World War II served a practical purpose: first and foremost it had to retain a woman's modesty, and also keep her warm – no wonder women's knickers were often referred to as 'passion killers'.

Knickers tended to be directoire/bloomer style (like a longer version of today's knickers with elasticated leg holes) or

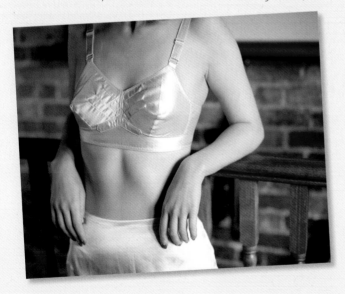

'French' knickers (like a female version of boxer shorts). French knickers were generally more popular and easier to obtain as they buttoned at the side and used very little, if any, elastic. They also required just two coupons, whereas a pair of directoire knickers needed three.

Bras underwent significant improvements during the 1930s, yet were not like the bras we wear today. They were soft and not underwired, normally made from rayon or silk (or sometimes crocheted). During the 1940s the bra was either worn as a separate piece or as part of a corselette – a full-length corset. Not everyone wore a brassiere. For many, especially working class girls, underwear consisted of knickers and some kind of vest/liberty bodice. An alternative was cami-knickers combining a camisole and knickers, which fastened under the crotch.

Ah stockings. When I think of 1940s fashion, stockings, or rather the lack of them, is one of the defining features. Stockings were often unattainable because silk, the main material used for them, was in short supply.

Above and right: Whilst original 1940s underwear can still be found, its sizes are out of sync with modern ones. Cup sizes in particular were still in their infancy in the 40s. I suggest trying repro brands to create the 40s shape underneath your clothes. What Katie Did make excellent repro French knickers and bras perfect for creating the 40s silhouette.

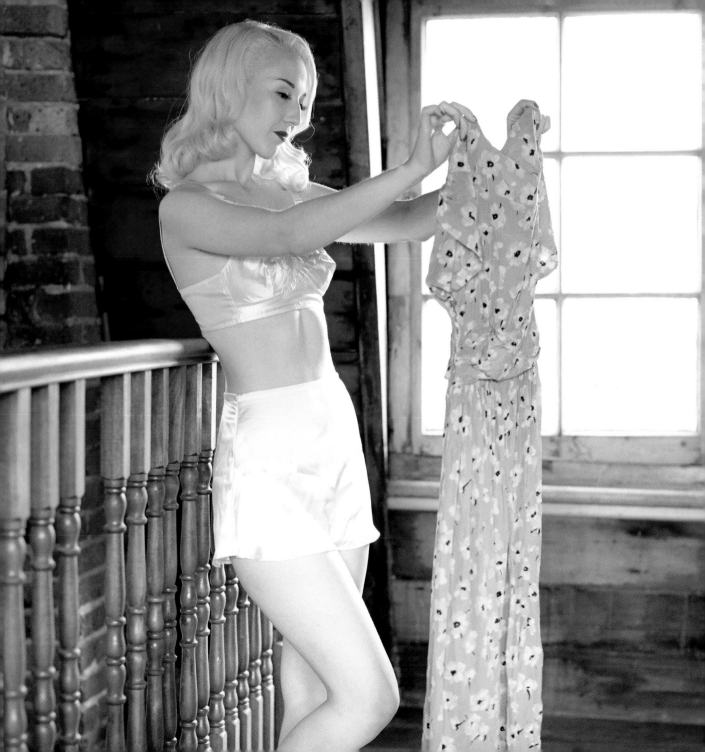

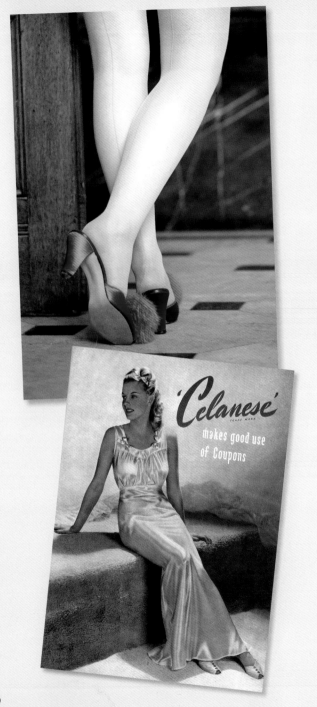

By the early 1940s there were alternatives to silk stockings on the market, the coveted American 'nylons'. In 1937 American firm DuPont patented nylon, and this was first used for stockings in 1939 (the first pairs went on sale in 1940). There was an insatiable desire for these new stockings in the USA and soon the news of them spread to the UK. Women acquired pairs either from generous GIs trying to woo them, or from relatives in America.

The scarcity of stockings left women with two options – either go stockingless, or use something to imitate the look of stockings. Some women covered their legs with gravy browning and drew on the stocking 'seam' with eyebrow pencil, but this attracted flies. It was also possible to purchase commercial paints known as 'liquid stockings' by the likes of Elizabeth Arden and Max Factor, but these ran if the wearer got wet or sweaty.

If a woman could acquire stockings they would be held up by suspenders, either on a belt or incorporated into a corset/corsolette.

Top left: Holly wears a pair of Daniel Green 1940s red satin mules with What Katie Did stockings. These are perfect for creating the 1940s look with their nude seam. For an authentic look seams should be nude or brown – other colours such as red were available during the 1940s, but they are rare finds.

Left: A Celanese (artificial silk) nightdress, 1944.

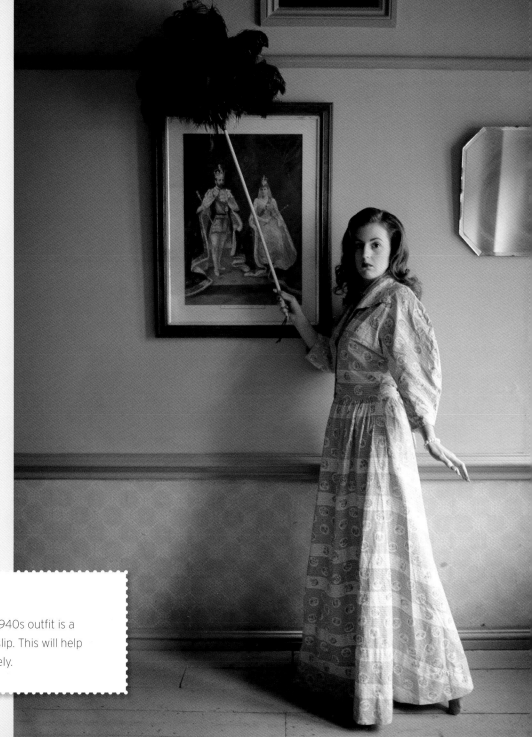

Right: Exuberant housecoats (like an indoor lounging dress) were fashionable throughout the 1940s – this example by Horrockses dates to 1948. During wartime these brightly coloured garments served a dual purpose – they were both attractive and warm. If one had to dash to an air raid shelter one could do so looking chic.

TOP TIP

An essential part of any 1940s outfit is a simple underskirt or full slip. This will help your skirt or dress sit nicely.

SWIMWEAR

By the 1940s swimwear as we recognise it today was coming into its own. There is something glamorous, chic and often escapist about swimwear during the 1940s. No longer were women restricted by heavy wool swimsuits that grew misshapen in water - increasingly swimwear was designed to show off a woman's curves.

In the USA during the war the beachwear industry (largely based around California and Portland, Oregon) was thriving. Swimwear was still being produced in Britain, but many lidos and outdoor pools were closed in order to conserve water.

As soon as the war was over the British public craved the beach and the lido more so than ever before. Many of my favourite family photographs show my Nanna, Great Aunt and their friends in 1946 and 1947 at the beach in their exuberant swimsuits and bikinis.

The end of the war saw major technological improvements in terms of swimwear. No longer were swimsuits produced only in cotton - now swimsuits were made using Lastex, nylon and other artificial fibres offering better fit and less loss of shape in water.

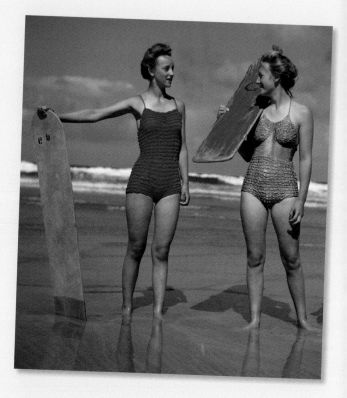

Above: British war workers take a seaside break on a beach in Cornwall, September 1943.

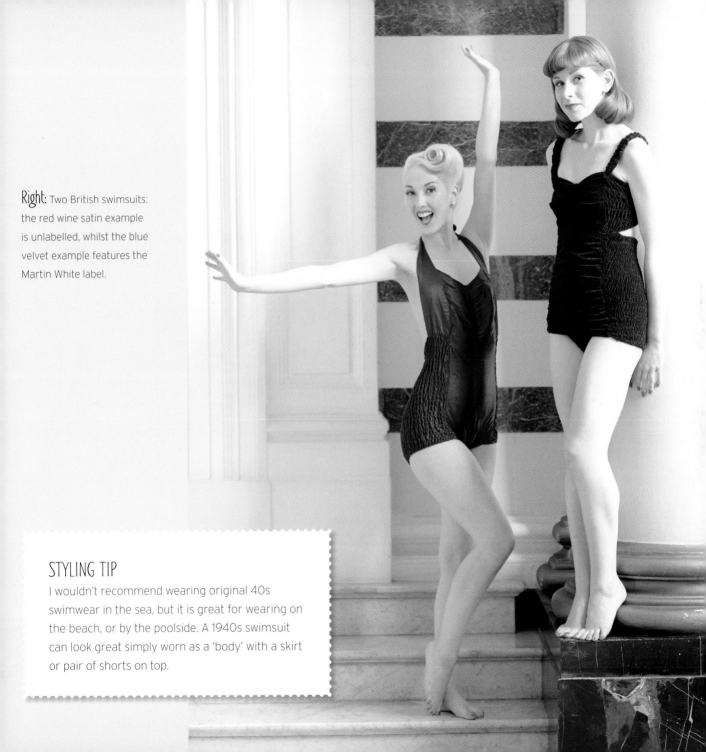

Right: Two British swimsuits: the red wine satin example is unlabelled, whilst the blue velvet example features the Martin White label.

STYLING TIP

I wouldn't recommend wearing original 40s swimwear in the sea, but it is great for wearing on the beach, or by the poolside. A 1940s swimsuit can look great simply worn as a 'body' with a skirt or pair of shorts on top.

THE BIKINI

Who 'invented' the bikini is one of those ubiquitous fashion questions that causes almost as much debate as who invented the miniskirt. In fact, two-piece swimsuits were seen on beaches and around swimming pools as early as the 1930s, but the term 'bikini' for the two-piece was not coined until 1946. Two Frenchmen Lluis Reard (an automotive engineer running his mother's lingerie business) and Jacques Heim (a Parisian couturier) created bikinis in 1946. What was novel about these suits was their skimpiness – they were navel-revealing, midriff-exposing creations. Heim's was what may now be viewed as a typical bikini, whereas Reard's was closer to what we may now call a string bikini.

Reportedly Reard's bikini was so tiny no Parisian model would agree to wear it! Micheline Bernadinini, a nude dancer at the Casino de Paris wore it for his first photoshoots. Heim christened his two-piece the 'atome' after the smallest known particle of matter. Reard called his the 'bikini' as the press conference for its launch was just five days after the first test of a nuclear device over the Bikini Atoll. Despite the fact that Reard's name stuck it was the styling of Heim's two-piece that gained popularity with the general public and became a swimwear fashion staple.

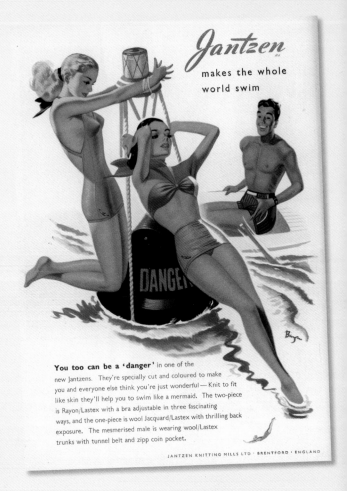

Jantzen makes the whole world swim

You too can be a 'danger' in one of the new Jantzens. They're specially cut and coloured to make you and everyone else think you're just wonderful — Knit to fit like skin they'll help you to swim like a mermaid. The two-piece is Rayon/Lastex with a bra adjustable in three fascinating ways, and the one-piece is wool Jacquard/Lastex with thrilling back exposure. The mesmerised male is wearing wool/Lastex trunks with tunnel belt and zipp coin pocket.

JANTZEN KNITTING MILLS LTD · BRENTFORD · ENGLAND

1940S SWIMWEAR LABELS TO LOOK OUT FOR
(many of these were still in operation after the 1940s!)

- Jantzen
- Martin White
- Catalina
- Cole of California
- Mallas Masllorens

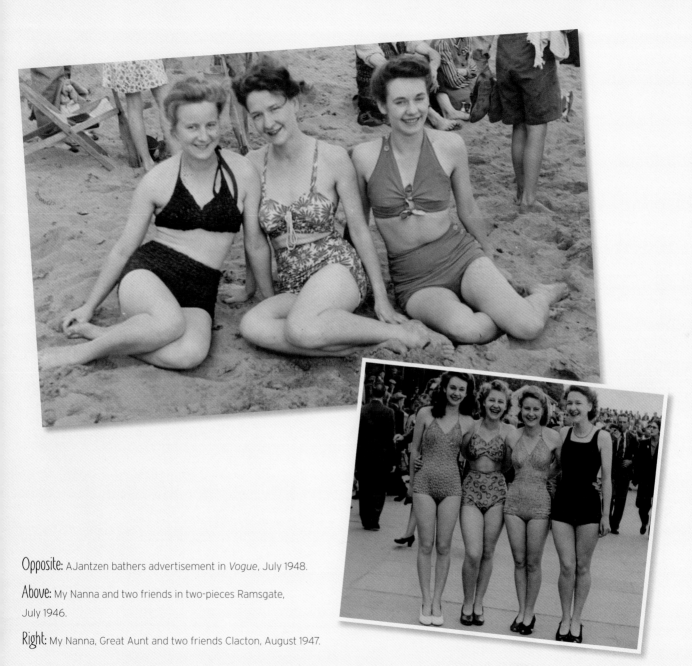

Opposite: A Jantzen bathers advertisement in *Vogue*, July 1948.

Above: My Nanna and two friends in two-pieces Ramsgate, July 1946.

Right: My Nanna, Great Aunt and two friends Clacton, August 1947.

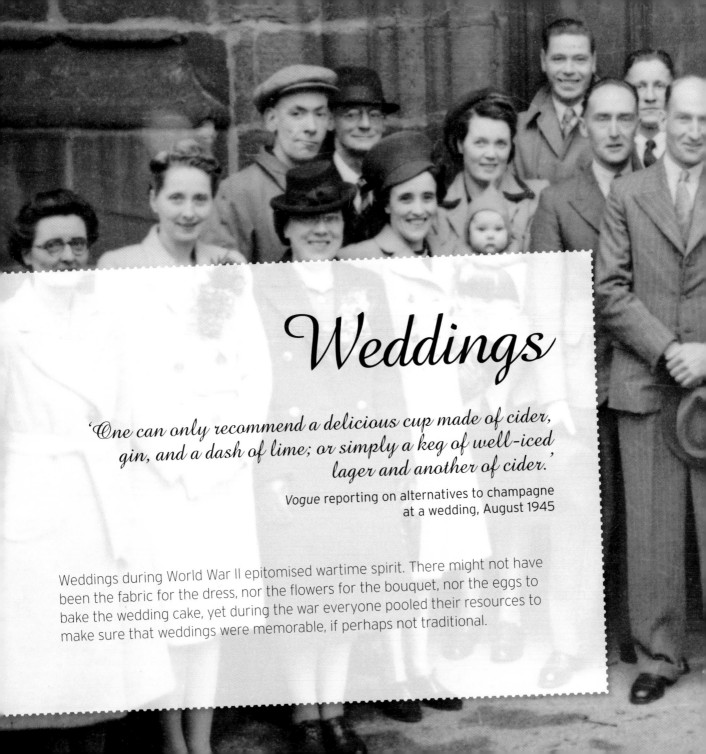

Weddings

'One can only recommend a delicious cup made of cider, gin, and a dash of lime; or simply a keg of well-iced lager and another of cider.'

Vogue reporting on alternatives to champagne
at a wedding, August 1945

Weddings during World War II epitomised wartime spirit. There might not have been the fabric for the dress, nor the flowers for the bouquet, nor the eggs to bake the wedding cake, yet during the war everyone pooled their resources to make sure that weddings were memorable, if perhaps not traditional.

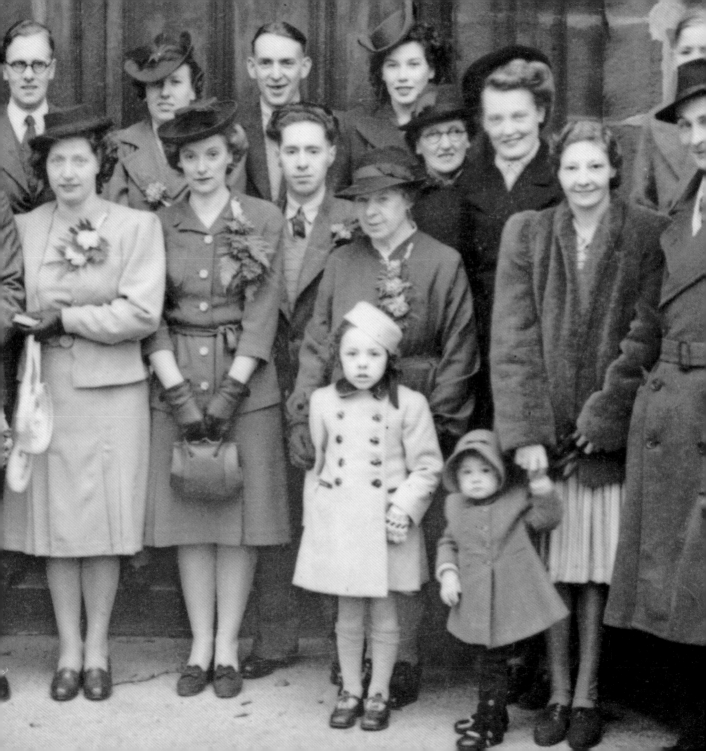

AND THE BRIDE WORE WHITE...
OR RED, OR BLUE, OR GREEN

Before 1939 most brides had a conventional wedding involving a church ceremony, white dress, bridesmaids and a reception to follow, but the war transformed this. One of the biggest changes was perhaps the planning of a wedding. Many married hastily and were given as little as 48 hours to prepare after receiving a telegram to say their fiancé was returning on leave. In situations such as these it was common for brides to borrow a dress or wear the smartest dress or suit that they already owned. Men on the other hand did not suffer such difficulties and the majority wore their service uniform for the ceremony.

Even for those with time to plan, the wartime wedding was a very different affair. Women were unwilling to spend coupons on a garment that would only be worn once. A neat suit or day dress was the choice for most brides.

For those who felt a white dress was a necessity it was possible to rent out wedding clothes. Moss Bros. who had being renting out men's wedding clothes since the 1890s, began to offer a similar service for brides.

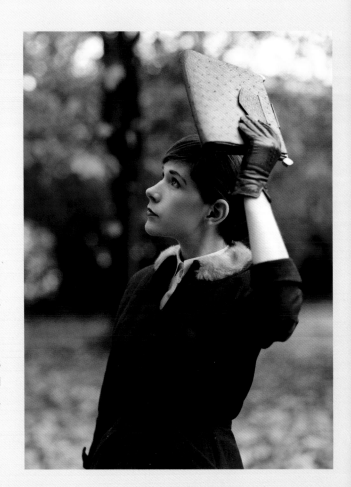

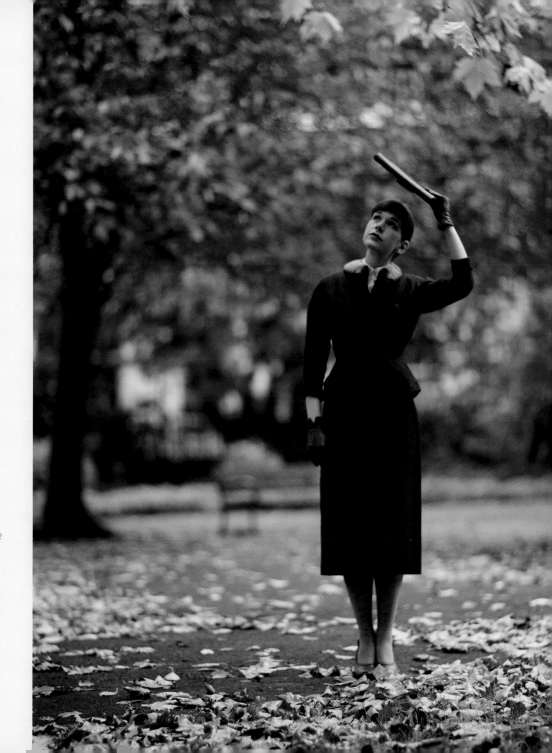

Left and right: This suit was originally worn as a going away outfit in 1948. It is made from wool and the collar is trimmed with mink. This demonstrates the other skirt style that was increasingly becoming popular in the late 1940s the long slim, almost pencil skirt. Again, this was a style popularised by Dior.

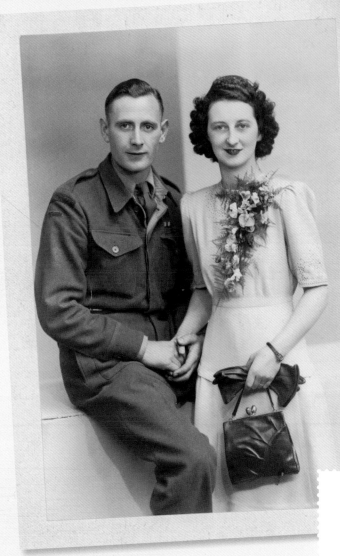

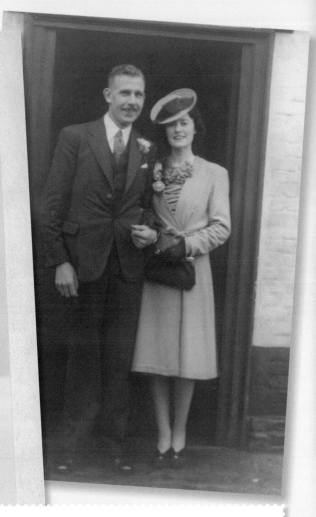

Above: The 1942 wedding of Herbert Hedges and Mavis. The bride wore a simple cream dress embellished with rhinestones and carried smart leather accessories.

TYPICAL WARTIME WEDDING LOOKS:

- Gathered sleeveheads
- Long sleeves
- V-shaped necklines
- Full length relatively narrow dresses
- Small corsage of flowers attached to the bride's dress
- Day dresses.

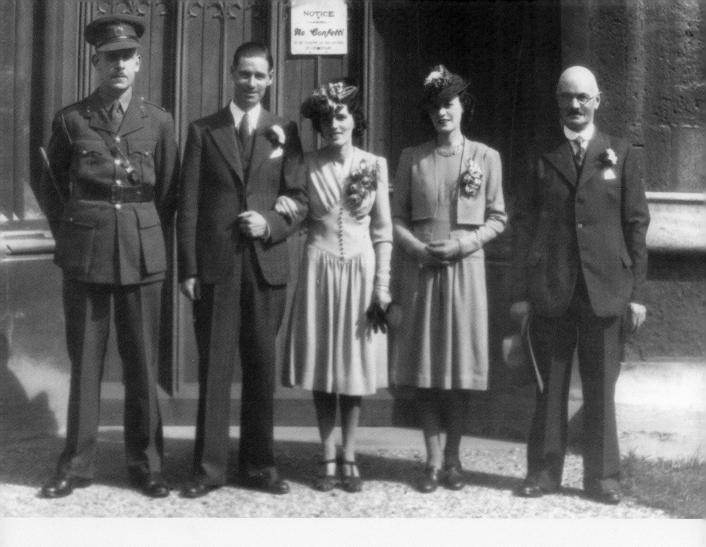

NOTICE.
No Confetti

Left: At this early 1940 wedding, the bride wore a blue suit with burgundy accessries. Again a corsage takes the place of a bouquet.

Floral decorations changed too. In the 1930s women had carried lavish and heavy bouquets, yet during the war women tended to carry a small posy of flowers, often picked from their garden with the addition of paper flowers, tulle or net to bulk it out.

Above: This December 1939 wedding of John Wilson to Gladys Hedges shows the move towards smart daywear as bridal attire.

Food shortages meant wedding receptions became far less lavish, and in many cases the bride and groom could not offer guests a meal. Wedding cakes were simpler affairs. Often cakes (owing to their meagre size) were covered with a cardboard icing that had to be lifted off to cut the cake.

THE AMERICANS HELP OUT THE BRITS

In 1943 Mrs John L Whitehurst, president of the General Federation of Women's Clubs, visited England and learnt that many girls were anxious to marry in the traditional white, but resources made it impossible. She decided to enlist American women to help and asked members of the GFWC to donate their wedding dresses. Fifty gowns were donated by American women for British servicewomen to wear. Each dress was loaned rather than given, to ensure that the dress would be worn by a number of brides until it was worn out.

Famous donors included Mary Pickford and Eleanor Roosevelt. Each gown had a little gold label providing the name and address of the dress donor. Many servicewomen suggested that this scheme was the only way that they had the opportunity to wear a white wedding dress.

The American wartime wedding was slightly different to the British one. Whilst women's clothing was restricted under L-85, wedding dresses were not included in the restrictions. American brides tended to still wear a traditional white dress. Very full skirts and long trains were rare finds though, and most dresses were made from rayon as opposed to silk.

The war created a more casual attitude to wedding attire and many women post war wore neat suits for their weddings. Especially in Britain, with rationing still in force, it was difficult to acquire a lavish dress. However, from 1946 onwards there were more cream and white wedding dresses available for the general public.

Right: This dress is one of my prized possessions. The original owner wore this for her wedding in 1948. Her family pooled together coupons so that she could purchase it. She wore the dress with a fine net veil embroidered with flowers and a pair of silk platform shoes by Lotus.

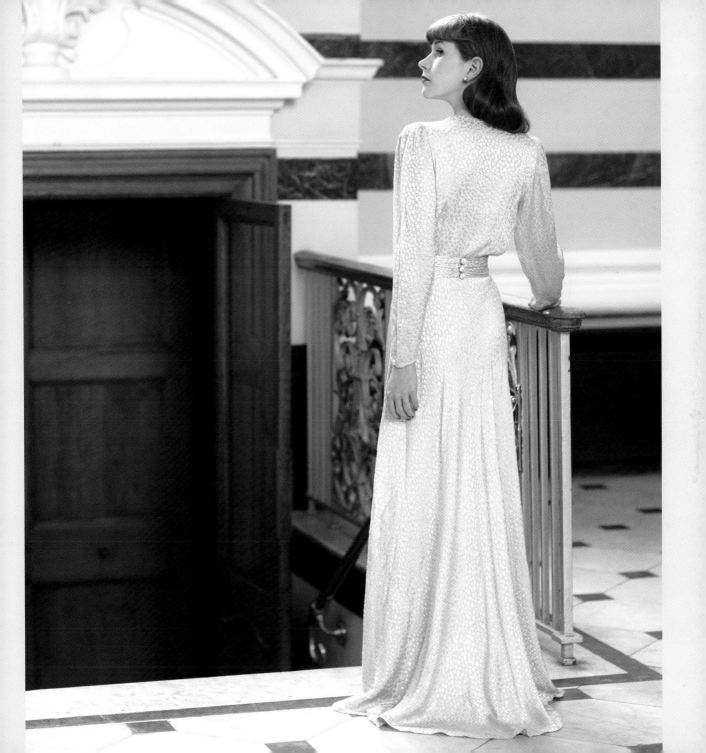

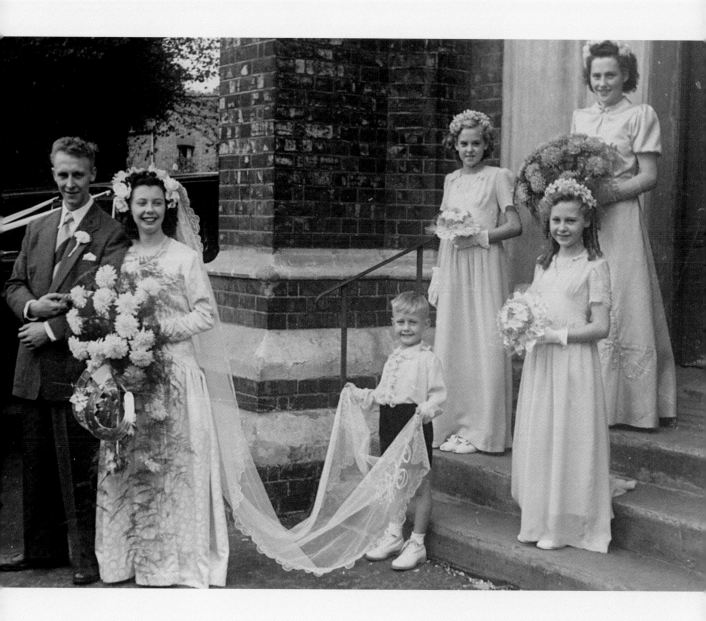

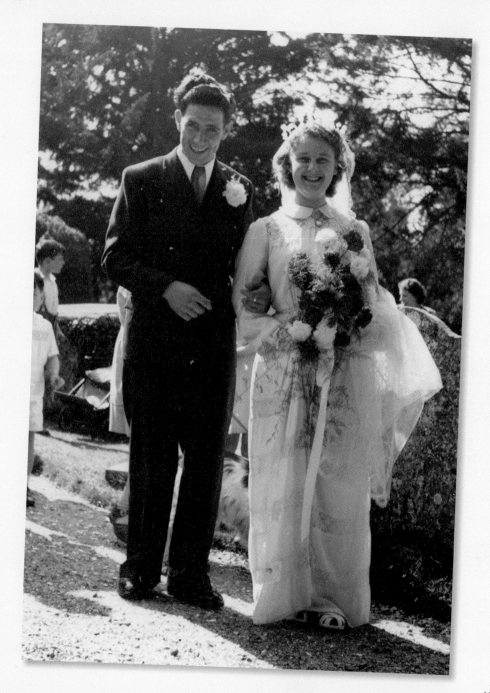

Left and right: Two 1948 weddings. My Great Aunt Rita (left) married in a full-length dress with long veil and huge bouquet, whilst my Great Aunt Thelma (right) married in a far simpler dress.

RESEARCHING THE 1940S

I am a total and utter research addict. When I'm not swishing around in vintage dresses you'll often find me holed up in a library with my nose deep in a musty copy of *Vogue*. Here are some of my favourite research resources to help you learn a little more about the 1940s.

FASHION MAGAZINES

Original 1940s magazines offer a unique insight into life during the war and immediately after. Comparing magazines from different countries also shows you quite how different life was from one country to another. Magazines such as *Vogue* illustrate how wealthier women dressed and lived their lives, whereas those such as *Modern Woman* (UK), *Good Housekeeping* (US and UK) and *Ladies Home Journal* (US) demonstrate how less affluent women lived.

Advertising space had to be cut and many British magazines were noticeably smaller in size during the war (*Vogue* for example had 100 pages during the war as opposed to 125 pages by 1948). British magazines were printed on thin, poor quality paper owing to paper rationing. When one compares a copy of American *Vogue* to British *Vogue* the difference is immediately evident. Printed on thick glossy paper, American *Vogue* was roughly one and a half times the size of the British issue!

Post war, every newspaper and magazine worth their salt carried a fashion column. One of my favourites is Alison Settle's (often very witty) column for the *Observer* ,'From a Woman's Viewpoint'. This offered Settle's opinions on the latest news in the fashion world.

Right: Keep your eyes peeled for wartime copies of British magazines - they are hard to come by and some, especially good condition copies of *Vogue*, command high sums.

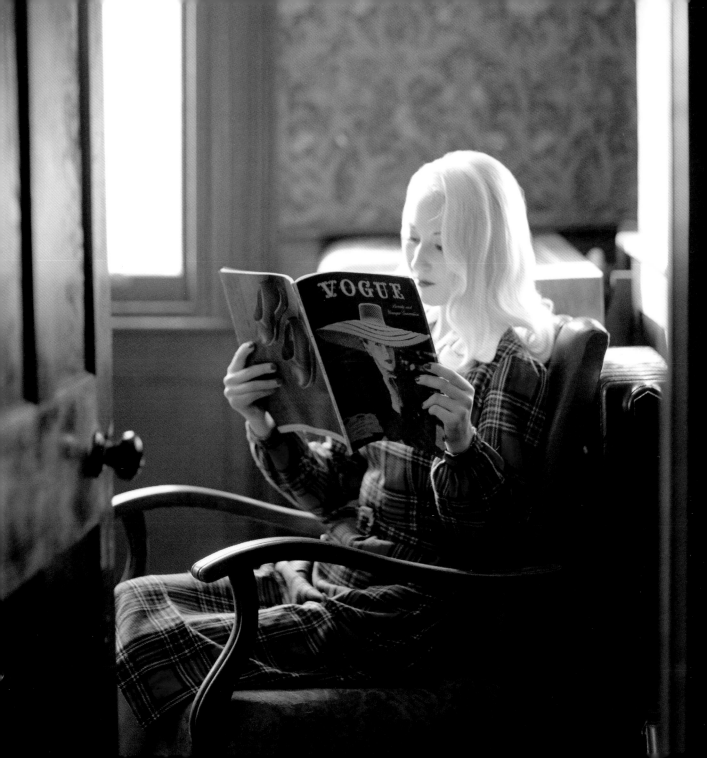

FILM

Another great tool for researching the 1940s are original films from the decade. Here are just a few of my top picks.

- *The Philadelphia Story* (1940) featuring Katharine Hepburn (opposite) in her iconic slacks.
- *Casablanca* (1942) A great watch for both Humphrey Bogart's classic trench coats and Ingrid Bergman's chic skirt suits.
- *Now Voyager* (1942) Bette Davis wears costumes by the Australian costume designer Orry-Kelly in this picture. Orry-Kelly was supposedly Davis's favourite costume designer.
- *Cabin In The Sky* (1943) MGM were considered to have taken a great risk with this film as it featured an unusual for the time all-African American cast.
- *Pin Up Girl* (1944) starring iconic wartime pin-up Betty Grable.
- *To Have And Have Not* (1944) The first film featuring the infamous Lauren Bacall and Humphrey Bogart coupling.
- *Cover Girl* (1944) A fabulous film featuring a selection of contemporary 1940s- and 1890s-inspired costumes.
- *The Big Sleep* (1946) Another classic Bogart and Bacall film with costumes by Leah Rhodes.
- *Gilda* (1946) A film noir featuring Rita Hayworth.
- *Key Largo* (1948) Lauren Bacall's appearance in this film wearing espadrilles apparently started the craze for them in America.
- *The Red Shoes* (1948) A definitive British film about a ballet dancer starring Moira Shearer.
- *Passport to Pimlico* (1949) A British Ealing comedy set during World War II.
- *Maytime in Mayfair* (1949) In my opinion one of the ultimate 1940s fashion films. Michael Gore-Brown (played by Michael Wilding) inherits a Mayfair dress shop.

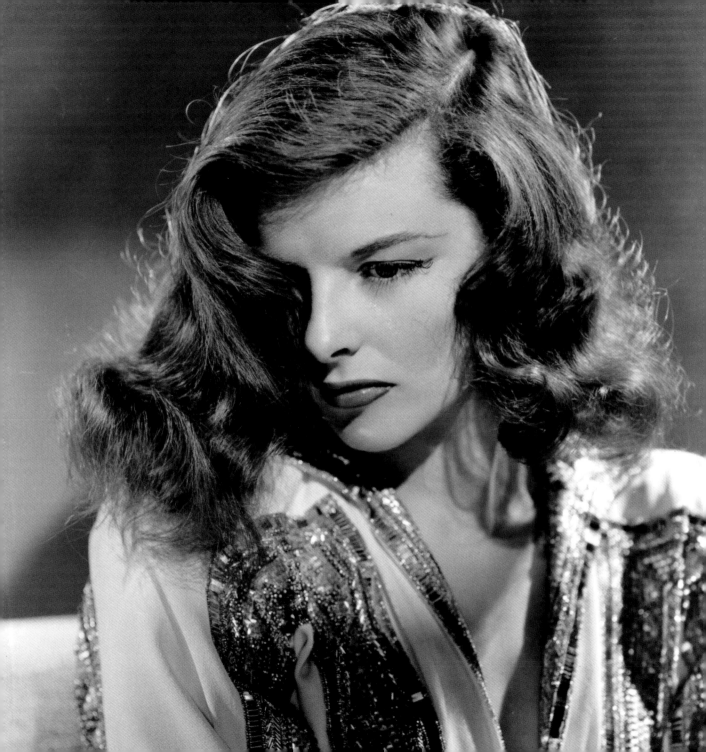

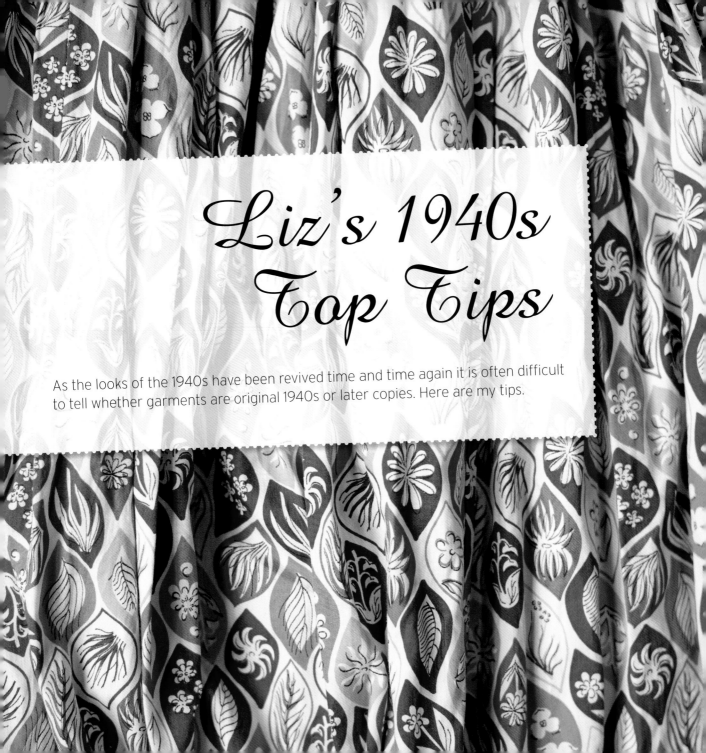

Liz's 1940s Top Tips

As the looks of the 1940s have been revived time and time again it is often difficult to tell whether garments are original 1940s or later copies. Here are my tips.

What sort of zip does the garment have? An original 1940s garment will likely have a metal zip (if it has one at all). It may also fasten with poppers at a side seam, or buttons. Later copies of 1940s garments are likely to have plastic zips. A common feature of 40s dresses (in particular American ones) is the double zip: a very short centre back zip at the neckline, and a long zip in the side seam.
What is the waistline like? Is it elasticated at all? An elasticated waistline normally indicates that a garment is 1970s or later.

How have the seams been finished? Are they overlocked? Overlocking is a strong sign of a garment from the 1960s or later.

What sort of labels does the garment have? Are there any care labels? Care labels featuring symbols were not mandatory in Britain until the early 1970s. Earlier pieces may have instructions on how to care for your garment, but no symbols will feature on them. Look out for brand labels too. Clothes of the 1940s often have elaborate labels with curling elegant script. Labels in 1940s garments can be hidden in strange places. If it hasn't got an immediately obvious label, turn it inside out to check side seams and waistbands.

What sort of shoulder pads does your garment have? A large and spongy-feeling shoulder pad is customarily a sign of a 1980s garment. 1940s shoulder pads tend to be harder and smaller.

What's the fabric like? Synthetic fabrics such as polyester indicate a later garment.

After you've handled a few original 1940s pieces it should become easier to identify them from later copies.

CARING FOR 1940S CLOTHES

- Watch out for rayon. Rayon is one of the most used 1940s fabrics, but it's difficult to care for. Rayon is prone to shrinking - whatever you do, don't put it in the washing machine! I highly recommend dry cleaning rayon, or you can hand wash in cold water with mild detergent.
- Be wary of cleaning sequinned garments. Gelatine sequins and beads will dissolve in water and melt under heat. If the beads on your garment are glass then it is fine to wash them.
- Store vintage knitwear flat to avoid it becoming misshapen.
- Deter moths with lavender sachets and cedar wood. Of the many things I've tried these seem to be the best option for keeping nasty critters at bay - and they keep your clothes smelling fresh!

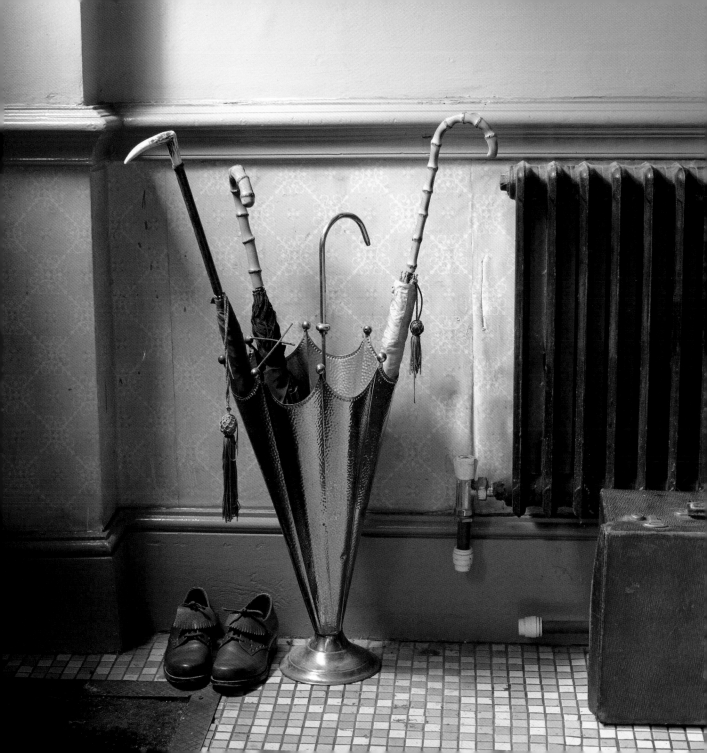

SHOPPING
1940S ORIGINALS

DARLINGS VINTAGE
www.etsy.com/shop/DarlingsVintageUK

DOROTHEA'S CLOSET
www.dorotheas-closet-vintage.myshopify.com

FABGABS
www.etsy.com/shop/FabGabs

GINGERMEGS
www.gingermegs-vintage.com

SCARLET RAGE
www.scarletragevintage.com

THE 40S ROOM
www.the40sroom.co.uk

THE VINTAGE AND REVIVAL CLOTHING COMPANY
www.vintage-revivalclothing.co.uk

VINTAGE HOARDS
www.etsy.com/shop/VintageHoards

UNIFORM HIRE

VINTAGE YEARS
www.costumehire.co.uk

Left: A tightly furled umbrella was the perfect finishing touch to the New Look.

1940S REPRODUCTION

If you love the 1940s look, but would prefer to buy new here are a few of my favourite brands that make the best reproduction and 1940s-inspired clothes and accessories.

Clothes

20TH CENTURY FOXY
www.20thcenturyfoxy.com

DELPHINE DELOVELY
www.facebook.com/DelphineDelovely

HEYDAY
www.heydayonline.co.uk

JITTERBUGGIN
www.etsy.com/shop/Jitterbuggin

KITTY LOU VINTAGE
www.etsy.com/shop/KittyLouVintage

MAIL ORDER PINUP
www.etsy.com/shop/MailOrderPinup

MISS BAMBOO
www.missbamboo.co.uk

MORELLOS
www.morellos.co.uk

NUDEEDUDEE
www.etsy.com/shop/nudeedudee

PUTTIN' ON THE RITZ
www.puttin-on-the-ritz.net

THE SEAMSTRESS OF BLOOMSBURY
www.theseamstressofbloomsbury.co.uk

SOMETHING ELSE CLOTHING
www.facebook.com/pages/Something-Else-Clothing

TRASHY DIVA
www.trashydiva.com

Reproduction WW2 uniforms

THE HISTORY BUNKER
www.thehistorybunker.co.uk

SOLDIER OF FORTUNE
www.sofmilitary.co.uk

APPLE TREE LANE
www.appletreelane.co.uk

Lingerie

WHAT KATIE DID
www.whatkatiedid.com

Jewellery

LUXULITE
www.etsy.com/shop/Luxulite

1940S STYLE FOR YOU
www.etsy.com/shop/1940sStyleForYou

Shoes

ARIS ALLEN
www.arisallen.com

JOHNSON SHOES
www.johnsonshoes.com

MISS L FIRE
www.misslfire.co.uk

REMIX
www.remixvintageshoes.com

ROCKET ORIGINALS
www.rocketoriginals.co.uk

Hats and Headpieces

ARTHELIA'S ATTIC
www.etsy.com/shop/ArtheliasAttic

B MILLINERY
www.bmillinery.com

BETSYHATTER
www.betsyhatter.co.uk

LADY EVE MILLINERY
www.etsy.com/shop/LadyEveMillinery

ROSIE ALIA
www.etsy.com/shop/RosieAliaDesigns

Right: Rosy wears a PinaFleur dress by Heyday. This modern dress is based on an original 1940s design.

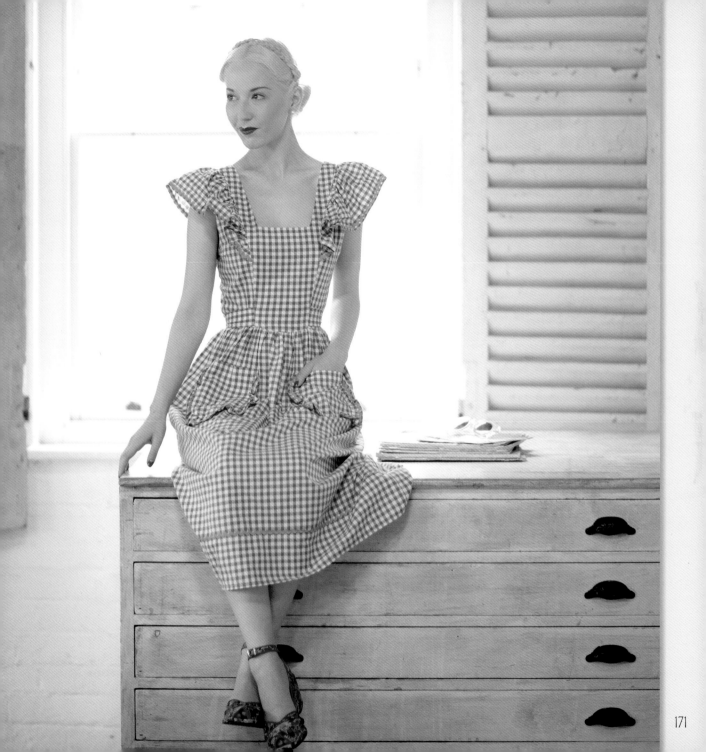

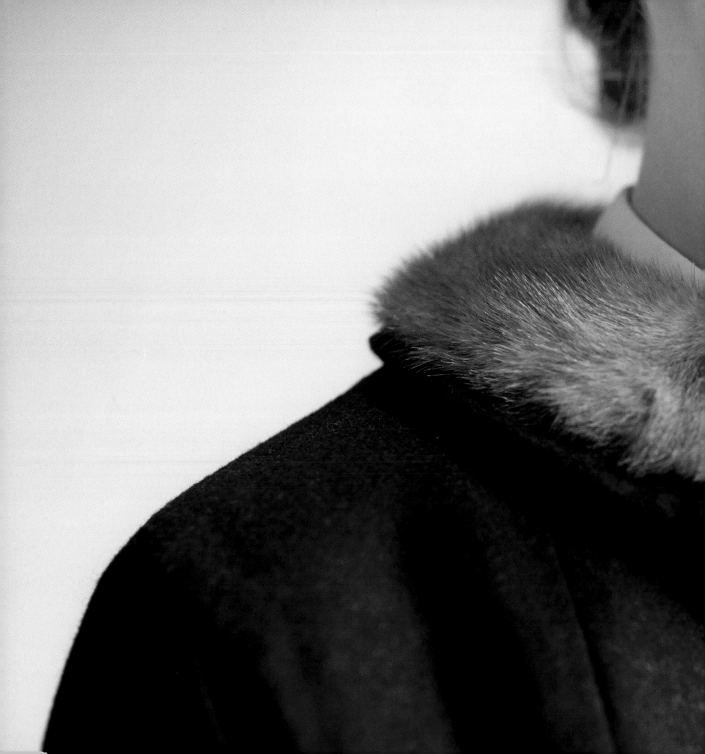

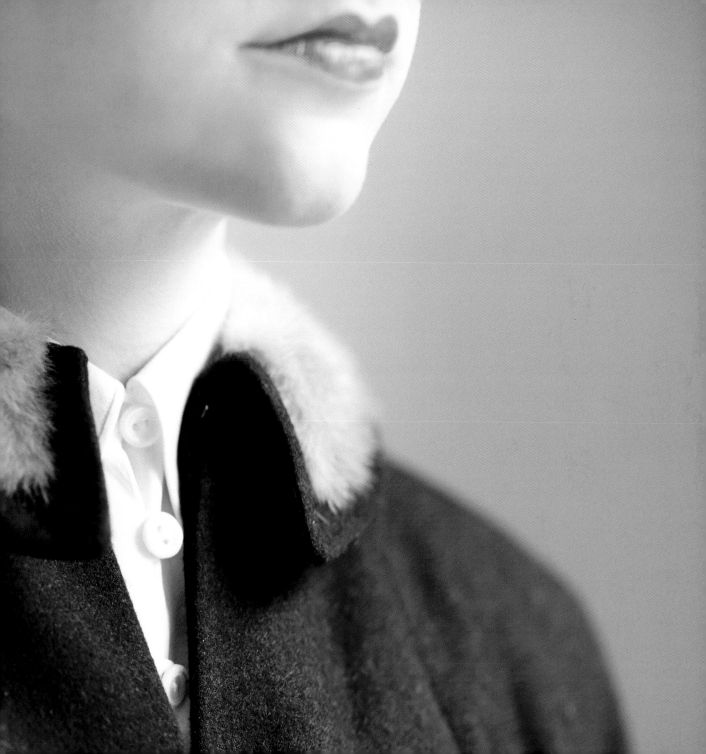

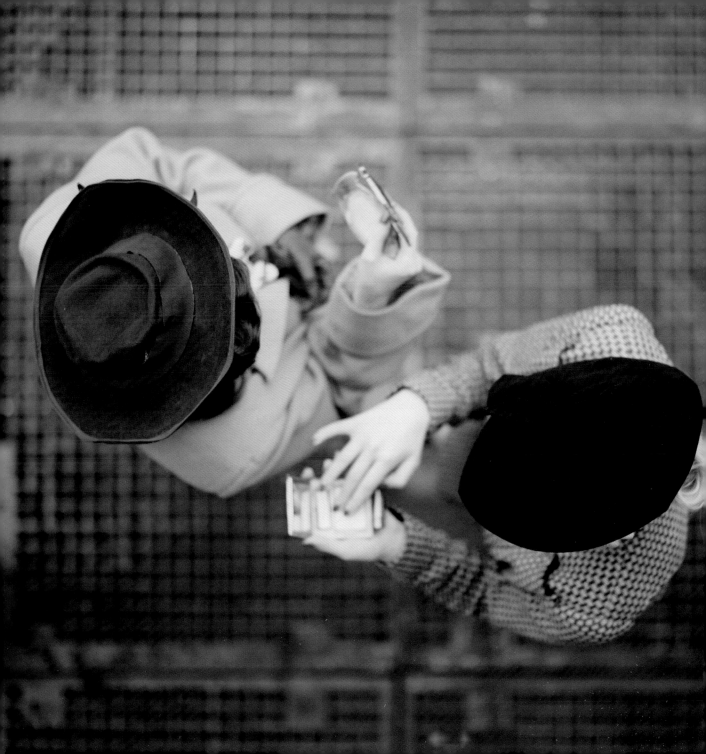

ACKNOWLEDGEMENTS AND THANKS

There are so many people I must say thank you to for helping me complete this book. Firstly my thanks must go to the numerous lovely people I know in the world of vintage. I must thank Rachel Wilkie not only for sending me so many pieces from her personal collection to use in the book but also for being a wonderfully supportive friend. Also a GIANT thank you to Jade Stavri for letting me raid both of her shops and also for just being such a crazy wonderful person. Thanks also go to the ladies who kindly lent pieces from their personal collections and shops- Ellie Thomas (I'm sure it was all for the incentive of kitty cuddles really), Ava Flynn, Alex Backhouse and Hadley Smythe. Thanks too to Shona Van Beers for lending the stunning Heyday PinaFleur dress and to Katy Crebbin for the amazing Luxulite jewellery.

The process of creating this book was made a joyful experience because of the fabulous team I worked with thank you to Rosy and Holly for being such wonderful models, and also a huge thanks to Natasha Hall for making them look so drop dead gorgeous. Brent Darby was just the best photographer, I love the humour you brought to our shoots. Thanks also to the assistants that worked with him- Kristy Noble and Claudia Moroni.

Thank you to Rebecca Winfield (www.davidluxtonassociates.co.uk) for being a wonderful agent (and for being a fantastic listener!) and to Emily Preece-Morrison at Pavilion Books for commissioning the book- I have loved working with you again!

Super special thanks to Naomi Thompson, without whom I doubt this book would ever have happened- you really are a one in a million friend.

I must also thank my wonderfully supportive and understanding boyfriend Martin – I am so sorry for the huge volume of 1940s 'stuff' that spent a few months living in our flat!

And finally thanks to my wonderful Nanna, Hazel Tregenza for sharing her stories and photographs with me. I couldn't have done it without you.

LOANS

Alex Backhouse **www.madamsvintage.com**
Katy Crebbin **www.etsy.com/shop/Luxulite**
Ava Flynn **www.etsy.com/shop/Veramode**
Hadley Smythe **www.hadleysmythe.com**
Jade Stavri **www.scarletragevintage.com**
Ellie Thomas **www.etsy.com/shop/DarlingsVintageUK**
Naomi Thomspon (and her Grandmother Margaret Chester!)
www.naomithompson.co.uk
Shona Van Beers **www.heyday.com**
Vintage years costume hire **www.costumehire.co.uk**
What Katie Did **www.whatkatiedid.com**
Rachel Wilkie **www.etsy.com/shop/VintageHoards**

HAIR AND MAKE-UP

Natasha Hall **www.prettymevintage.co.uk**

MODELS

Holly Foster **www.secretdreamworldofavintagegirl.blogspot.co.uk**
Rosy Apples **www.facebook.com/RosyApples**

First published in the United Kingdom in 2015 by
Pavilion Books Company Ltd
1 Gower Street, London WC1E 6HD

Commissioning editor: Emily Preece-Morrison
Designer: Briony Hartley
Photographer: Brent Darby

ISBN: 9781909815933

A CIP catalogue record for this book is available from the British Library.

Colour reproduction by Rival Colour Ltd., UK
Printed and bound by 1010 Printing International Ltd., China

This book can be ordered direct from the publisher at
www.pavilionbooks.com

10 9 8 7 6 5 4 3 2 1

PICTURE CREDITS

All special photography by Brent Darby except those credited below.
©: p. 6: Liz Tregenza; p.7: PF-(bygone1) / Alamy; p.12: Jeff Morgan 02 / Alamy; p.13: Moviepix / Getty; p.14: Mary Evans Picture Library / Alamy; p.27: Antiques & Collectables / Alamy; p.30: Moviepix / Getty; p.31: Moviepix / Getty; p32T: Imperial War Museums; p.32B: Liz Tregenza; p.40: The LIFE Picture Collection / Getty; p.46T and B: PF-(bygone1) / Alamy; p.53: Liz Tregenza; p.55: Imperial War Museums; p.57: Imperial War Museums; p.59: Hulton Archive / Getty; p.60: Imperial War Museums; p.68: Imperial War Museums; p.70: Imperial War Museums; p.72: The Lucinda Moore Collection / Mary Evans; p.74: Liz Tregenza; p.76L and R: The National Army Museum / Mary Evans Picture Library; p.77: Heritage Image Partnership Ltd / Alamy; pp.78-9: National Film Board of Canada / Getty; p.84: IWM/Getty Images; p.96: Gamma-Keystone / Getty; pp.98-9: Hulton Archive / Getty; p.101 Hulton Archive / Getty; p.105: Picture Post / Getty; p.106: Mary Evans/Epic/Tallandier; p.110: Liz Tregenza; p.112L: Liz Tregenza; p112R: Hulton Archive / Getty; p.113: Liz Tregenza; p.128: Photos 12 / Alamy; p.130: Glasshouse Images / Mary Evans; p.138: Mary Evans Picture Library/LESLEY BRADSHAW; p.146B: Mary Evans Picture Library; p.148: Popperfoto / Getty; p.150: Mary Evans Picture Library; p.151T and B: Liz Tregenza; p.152-3: Mary Evans Picture Library/JJT; p.156L and R: Emily Morrison; p.157: Emily Morrison; p.160: Liz Tregenza; p.161: Liz Tregenza; p.165: Moviepix / Getty Images.

ALSO AVAILABLE FROM PAVILION BOOKS:

Liz Tregenza is a vintage fashion specialist and historian, and recently graduated with a Masters in Design History from the RCA. Liz has worked for a number of museums including Hampshire museums service and the V&A. She co-curated her first museum show at the age of 20 and has since contributed to numerous books and research papers. Liz is an avid collector of all things novelty.